THE SIMPLE MENOPAUSE MANUAL

A HOLISTIC APPROACH TO MANAGE HOT FLASHES,
CONTROL WEIGHT GAIN, AND GET OFF THE
HORMONE ROLLERCOASTER WITH EASE

MAX HAMPTON

CONTENTS

INTRODUCTION

The journey through menopause can often feel like stepping onto an uncharted path. Whether you're suddenly hit with hot flashes, experiencing unexpected mood swings, or realizing that your body is entering a new phase of life, the first encounters with menopause can be both daunting and bewildering.

I've witnessed this firsthand—in the faces of friends, the experiences of women in my community, and especially in my partner's struggles. Every woman's story is unique, but they all share a common thread: the need for understanding, guidance, and support.

Our journey begins here. Menopause isn't a time of loss or decline but an opportunity for an exciting new adventure. It's an invitation to rediscover ourselves, reconnect with our bodies, and enhance our overall well-being. As with any adventure, having a reliable guide can make all the difference, and that's where this book comes in.

This manual is more than just a guide; it's your companion through the changes that come with menopause. It offers holistic strategies to manage hot flashes, weight gain, and the hormone rollercoaster. It's a companion to support, empower, and help you take control of your well-being.

This journey isn't just about managing symptoms or getting through menopause. It's about embracing the adventure, cherishing the experience, and nurturing your health every step of the way. Together, we'll explore this new terrain, and I'll ensure you're well-prepared to navigate it with ease, wisdom, and a sense of empowerment.

Let's begin our adventure together. Welcome to the Simple Menopause Manual.

1

THE MENOPAUSE MAP

Have you ever found yourself standing at the entrance of a labyrinth, peering into the intricate maze before you, wondering where to begin? Metaphorically speaking, the onset of menopause might feel the same— like navigating a complex maze filled with twists and turns, where every route seems to lead to a dead-end.

But here's the thing: every maze has an exit, a way out, a path that takes you to the other side. With the proper understanding and knowledge, you can find your way through the menopause maze and emerge on the other side victorious and empowered.

DEFINING THE LANDSCAPE: WHAT IS MENOPAUSE?

Menopause is a natural process that every woman goes through. It marks the end of her reproductive years when the ovaries stop releasing eggs, leading to the discontinuation of menstrual cycles. However, menopause is not just about periods stopping; it's a complex hormonal shift that impacts almost every aspect of a woman's life.

This transformative phase, usually occurring in a woman's late 40s or early 50s, is characterized by a decline in the production of estrogen and progesterone—two vital hormones governing the female reproductive system. The fluctuating hormonal levels can induce a variety of physical and emotional changes. Common symptoms include hot flashes, night sweats, mood swings, and vaginal dryness, which can lead to discomfort and affect a woman's quality of life.

But menopause's effects go beyond physical health. It can have a significant impact on a woman's emotional well-being and relationships. Hormonal imbalances can lead to feelings of anxiety, depression, and irritability, straining both intimate and familial relationships.

The journey through menopause also raises long-term health concerns. The loss of estrogen's protective effects on bones and blood vessels can increase the risk of conditions like osteoporosis and cardiovascular disease. This makes it crucial for women to prioritize their overall health through a balanced diet, regular exercise, and discussions with healthcare professionals about potential hormone replacement therapy or other treatments.

Biological Transition

Biology and nature are filled with transitions, like a caterpillar transforming into a butterfly or a seed sprouting into a plant. Menopause is one such natural metamorphosis, signaling the start of a new phase of life.

Just like a seedling needs the right conditions to flourish, understanding the biological changes happening in your body can better equip you to navigate menopause confidently.

Hormonal Shifts

Estrogen and progesterone are the stars of the show when it comes to menopause. These hormones have been a part of your life since puberty, regulating everything from your menstrual cycle to your mood. As you approach menopause, their production starts to decline, triggering a range of physical and emotional changes.

Think of it like a see-saw. During your reproductive years, estrogen and progesterone are in perfect balance, working harmoniously to regulate your menstrual cycle. As menopause approaches, this balance is disrupted. The see-saw tips, setting off changes throughout your body.

It's a bit like adjusting to a new climate after a big move. At first, the heat or cold might seem overwhelming, but with time, your body gets used to the new conditions. Similarly, while the hormonal shifts of menopause might feel disruptive initially, understanding these changes can help you manage the transition more effectively.

End of Fertility

Menopause marks the end of a woman's ability to conceive naturally. This momentous milestone can evoke a range of emotions. For some women, it might bring a sense of relief, especially if childbearing years were marked by painful periods or fertility challenges. For others, menopause might trigger feelings of loss or sadness.

Regardless of the emotions this new life stage stirs up, the end of fertility is a significant aspect of menopause. It's a reminder that our bodies are continually evolving, and each life stage brings unique challenges and joys.

Like a gardener tending to the soil and sowing seeds, caring for your body during menopause is vital to your overall well-being. Understanding the biological transition, hormonal shifts, and the end of fertility that define menopause is the first step in this process.

Consider this your guidebook—your manual for the menopause journey. It's designed to provide you with the knowledge and tools you need to navigate the maze of menopause confidently. While the path may be filled with twists and turns, remember that every maze has an exit, a way out. With the right understanding, you can find your way and emerge on the other side victorious and empowered.

As we delve deeper into the world of menopause, remember that knowledge is power. The more you understand about your body and the changes it's going through, the better prepared you'll be to manage the transition effectively. You are not alone on this journey. With every page you read, you'll discover understanding, guidance, and support to help you confidently navigate the maze of menopause.

THE MENOPAUSE TRANSITION: KNOWLEDGE FOR EMPOWERMENT AND WELLNESS

Every woman will eventually go through menopause, underscoring the significance of being well-informed and prepared for this natural phase. Recognizing this need, educational institutions have incorporated menopause education into their curriculums since September 2020. It's essential to understand the changes your body goes through as you wrap up your reproductive years and stop menstruating.

Menopause is a noteworthy chapter in a woman's life, and getting familiar with it in advance can promote a sense of readiness and comfort. This book explores the various changes that come with menopause, such as joint pain, vaginal dryness, fatigue, hair loss, and psychological shifts that can influence one's well-being.

Many women have shared that their experiences of menopause have been challenging, often attributing these difficulties to a lack of knowledge and preparation. By introducing this subject to young girls and women who have not yet reached this stage of life, we can instill a sense of empowerment and support as they approach and navigate this significant life transition.

POSTMENOPAUSAL ZEST: CULTIVATING OPTIMISM BEYOND MENOPAUSE

Menopause, often perceived as a challenging time, can also be a period of significant personal growth and empowerment. The idea of "postmenopausal zest" reflects the renewed enthusiasm for life many women experience after menopause. Anthropologist Margaret Mead once noted the remarkable energy of postmenopausal women, and research has shown that this period of time can be marked by increased optimism, creativity, and emotional well-being.

Susan Feldman, the founder of Get in the Groove, speaks to the emotional freedom and resilience that can come with age, highlighting the shift in perspective and the strength to prioritize personal goals that often emerge after menopause. Dr. Heather Silvestri, a psychologist, echoes this sentiment, suggesting that the transition is a natural turning point for women, allowing them to shape their postmenopausal lives with openness and curiosity. Self-care techniques like regular exercise, gratitude practices, and mindfulness can greatly enhance this experience.

The Association for Women's Health Care also offers practical advice for women navigating menopause and encourages a proactive approach to maintaining a healthy lifestyle. A balanced diet rich in nutrients can support bone health. At the same time, regular exercise can improve both physical and mental well-being. Additionally, staying hydrated, following a consistent sleep pattern, and seeking treatments as needed, including hormone replacement therapy for symptom management, can contribute to a positive menopause experience.

By combining a positive and constructive attitude with lifestyle adjustments and self-care, the transition through menopause can become an empowering and fulfilling phase of life. This approach not only benefits the individual but can also influence societal perspectives on menopause, promoting a more positive and respectful understanding of this natural life stage.

THE THREE STAGES: PERIMENOPAUSE, MENOPAUSE, AND POSTMENOPAUSE

Menopause is not a single event but a series of stages that unfold over time. Think about this progression through perimenopause, menopause, and postmenopause like acts in a play, each with its unique characteristics and experiences.

Perimenopause: The Prelude

The curtain lifts with perimenopause, which is the prelude to the main event. This life stage can start up to ten years before menopause and is characterized by a gradual decline in estrogen production.

Picture a summer day slowly fading into evening, the light gradually diminishing. That's perimenopause. You might not notice the changes at first, but as you inch closer to menopause, the signs become more noticeable. You might experience irregular periods, hot flashes, sleep disturbances, or mood swings. But remember, like the evening slowly giving way to night, these changes are a natural part of the transition.

Menopause: The Main Event

Following perimenopause is menopause, which is the main event. This stage is marked by the absence of menstrual periods for 12 consecutive months. The spotlight here is on the ovaries as they retire from their job of releasing eggs and producing most of your estrogen.

Think of this stage like a seasoned actress taking her final bow on stage, signaling the end of an era. This shift can bring a host of symptoms, including hot flashes, night sweats, and vaginal dryness. But just as the applause recognizes the actress's contribution, understanding these symptoms can help you appreciate your body's hard work and resilience.

Postmenopause: The Aftermath

Postmenopause, the aftermath, is the stage that follows menopause, where symptoms like hot flashes gradually decrease and your body adjusts to its new hormonal environment.

Imagine a theater after the final act of a play. The audience departs, the lights dim, and a calm settles over the stage. That's postmenopause. The climatic symptoms of menopause recede, and a new normal sets in. This phase can last for the rest of your life, and while the symptoms of menopause usually decrease, long-term effects of lowered estrogen levels, like bone loss, may begin to surface.

This three-act play of menopause might seem daunting, but understanding each phase of the transition can equip you with the knowledge you need to navigate the journey. It's like having a map for a labyrinth—with understanding, you can anticipate turns and avoid dead-ends. As we explore further, remember that while menopause may be a universal experience, every woman's journey is unique. Your experience will be shaped by your body, health, and lifestyle choices.

Armed with this knowledge, you're now well-prepared to navigate the maze of menopause. Let's move forward not with trepidation but with the confidence that comes from understanding. The labyrinth of menopause may be complex, but remember, every maze has a path that leads to the other side. You're not alone on this journey, and with each step you take, you'll find the knowledge and tools you need to navigate this life stage with ease and empowerment.

THE HORMONE ROLLER COASTER: ESTROGEN AND PROGESTERONE

Menopause, in its essence, is a hormonal shift—a roller-coaster ride where the levels of two key hormones, estrogen and progesterone, fluctuate and eventually decline. Understanding these hormones, their roles, and their interplay can help you navigate this journey more effectively.

Estrogen's Role

Estrogen, often known as the 'female' hormone, is the star of the hormonal cast. Its responsibilities are wide-ranging and essential. From regulating the menstrual cycle to maintaining bone density and keeping your skin supple, estrogen is a valuable player in women's health.

Think of estrogen as the conductor of an orchestra. It directs and coordinates various instruments, ensuring that every member plays in harmony. When estrogen levels are balanced, the body functions like a well-tuned orchestra, with each system playing its part in perfect harmony.

During menopause, however, estrogen production declines, disrupting this harmony. The result can be a range of symptoms, from hot flashes to mood swings. It's similar to an orchestra playing without a conductor, resulting in a cacophony rather than a symphony. By understanding estrogen's role, you can better predict and manage these changes.

Progesterone's Part

If estrogen is the orchestra's conductor, progesterone is the sheet music. This hormone plays a supporting but crucial role in women's health. It prepares your body for pregnancy each month and regulates menstruation. It's also a natural balancer for estrogen, maintaining a delicate hormonal equilibrium.

During menopause, progesterone levels decrease along with estrogen. This decline can disrupt the hormonal balance, contributing to symptoms like irregular periods and sleep disturbances. It's as if the sheet music got lost along the way, throwing the orchestra into disarray. Recognizing progesterone's part in this hormonal maze can help you make sense of the changes you're experiencing.

The Balancing Act

The relationship between estrogen and progesterone is a delicate one. When in harmony, these hormones support optimal health and well-being. However, during menopause, this balance is disrupted, leading to various physical and emotional symptoms.

Imagine a tightrope walker maintaining perfect balance. This is similar to your body during your reproductive years, with estrogen and progesterone working in perfect harmony. Menopause, however, is like a gust of wind disrupting the tightrope walker's balance. The resulting wobble is a normal response, and understanding this disruption can help you better navigate the transition to menopause.

Menopause is more than hormonal shifts; it's a phase of adaptation and transformation. While the decline in estrogen and progesterone may trigger a range of symptoms in your mind and body, it's essential to remember that these changes are a normal part of the transition.

Understanding the roles of estrogen and progesterone, as well as the balancing act between them, is an essential step in navigating menopause. It provides a roadmap—a guide to the hormonal shifts that define this phase. It helps you to understand your body better, manage your symptoms, and ultimately, navigate the maze of menopause with confidence.

As we continue to explore the journey of menopause, remember that knowledge is your compass. It illuminates the path ahead, guiding you through the twists and turns of the menopause maze. So, now that we are better equipped with the understanding and tools to navigate this transition confidently and easily, let's press on.

While menopause may be a complex maze, you can be confident that with the right knowledge, you can find your way out on the other side. You're not alone on this journey. Each step takes you closer to the exit, to the other side of the maze of menopause. And with every page you turn in this guide, you'll find more knowledge, tools, and confidence to navigate this transition with ease and empowerment.

So, let's continue with confidence, leaving behind fear and anxiety. While menopause may seem like a complex maze, remember that every maze has an exit. With every step you take, you're getting close to finding your way out. The journey through menopause may be challenging, but you're not alone. With understanding, support, and guidance, you can navigate this transition with confidence, ease, and empowerment.

MENOPAUSE TIMELINE: WHAT TO EXPECT WHEN

Mapping the journey through menopause can be compared to forecasting the weather. There are patterns and rhythms, clear indicators of what's to come, but there's also a degree of unpredictability and a unique variability that makes each woman's experience distinctly her own.

Early Signs

Early signs of menopause often appear during perimenopause, and they can be subtle, like the first light of dawn breaking the night's darkness. You might notice shifts in your menstrual cycle, with periods becoming irregular or changing in intensity. Some women might also experience hot flashes—those sudden, transient waves of heat that can leave you flushed and sweating.

Mood swings might also make an entrance, which are a rollercoaster of emotions that can feel somewhat disturbing, similar to the mood changes you may have experienced during premenstrual syndrome (PMS) in your younger years. Additionally, sleep may become elusive or disturbed, like trying to catch a butterfly in the wind.

The early signs of menopause are your body's way of signaling change, much like leaves changing color in the fall. It's an announcement of a new season, a transition that, while sometimes challenging, is a natural part of life's ebb and flow.

Peak Symptoms

As menopause approaches, the symptoms often intensify, reaching their peak. This is your body's adaptation to a new rhythm—a new hormonal balance. Hot flashes, like an unexpected summer heatwave, may become more frequent or intense.

Sleep disturbances might persist, making falling or staying asleep more difficult. It might feel like insomnia, where sleep is a distant dream. Vaginal dryness may make an appearance as well, often accompanied by a loss of libido. Weight gain, particularly around the abdomen, might also be noticeable, like a favorite pair of jeans suddenly fitting a little too snug.

During this time, it's essential to remember that it's okay to seek help and to reach out to healthcare professionals, friends, or support groups. Much like a mountain climber uses safety ropes and harnesses, having a support system during this life stage can provide the necessary safety and assurance during this challenging climb.

Post-Menopause Changes

As you transition into post-menopause, the hot flashes and night sweats typically subside like a storm passing and leaving behind a calm sky. However, this stage has its challenges.

Decreased estrogen levels might lead to long-term changes like loss of bone density, increasing the risk of osteoporosis. It's similar to the thinning of an eggshell; it's a subtle yet significant change. Additionally, changes to cardiovascular health may occur, emphasizing the importance of a heart-healthy lifestyle.

The postmenopausal stage, while presenting its unique challenges, also ushers in a new phase of life: a time of self-discovery and growth. It's a testament to your body's resilience—a badge of honor that speaks of the journey you've navigated.

While each woman's menopause timeline is unique, understanding the expected progression can give you a better sense of control and preparedness. It equips you with the knowledge to recognize and understand the changes, empowering you to take proactive steps toward managing your symptoms and maintaining your overall well-being.

Menopause, while a significant life transition, is not a destination; instead, it's a pathway to a new phase of life and a testament to your body's resilience and strength. It's a reminder of life's cyclical nature and the ebb and flow of seasons. As you continue to navigate this stage, remember that every challenge presents an opportunity for growth, every symptom is a signal of change, and every change is a step towards a new equilibrium. Menopause is not an end but a beginning. It's a gateway to a new phase of life that holds the promise of growth, empowerment, and discovery.

Checklist: Symptoms to Observe

Please check any symptoms you've experienced in the past month:

- Irregular periods
- Hot flashes
- Night sweats
- Sleep disturbances
- Mood swings
- Vaginal dryness
- Decrease in libido
- Dry skin
- Thinning hair
- Weight gain

Note: Not everyone will experience all of these symptoms, and some might experience others not listed. This checklist is just a starting point.

Interactive Element: Test Your Knowledge

Answer the following questions to see how well you understand menopause.

1. What is menopause?

    A) The process of aging
    B) The end of monthly menstrual cycles
    C) The time when women experience intense PMS
    D) The onset of menstrual cycles during puberty

2. Which hormone levels drop during menopause?

    A) Testosterone
    B) Insulin
    C) Estrogen and progesterone
    D) Adrenaline

3. At approximately what age does perimenopause typically start?

    A) Late 20s
    B) Late 30s to early 40s
    C) Early 50s
    D) Late 60s

Answers: 1-B, 2-C, 3-B

To-Do: Time to Reflect

Take a moment to reflect:

- Write down any instances in the past year where you've felt changes in your body that might be related to menopause.
- Consider discussing these changes with someone you trust— this could be a friend, family member, or your doctor.
- Research any symptoms or experiences you're unsure about to gain a better understanding.
- Schedule a dedicated time each week to check in with yourself, noting any new or recurring symptoms.

2

SYMPTOMS AND SOLUTIONS

P icture stepping outside into a winter's chill, only to be engulfed by a sudden and intense heat as if you've been thrust into a midsummer heatwave. This abrupt and unexpected sensation is what many women experience during hot flashes, which is one of the most common symptoms of menopause. Just as each woman's experience with menopause is unique, so too is the way her body communicates these changes. In this chapter, we will focus on decoding this language, beginning with exploring hot flashes and night sweats.

HOT FLASHES AND NIGHT SWEATS: YOUR BODY'S NEW LANGUAGE

Hot flashes and night sweats can make you feel like your body is speaking a foreign language. But with patience and understanding, you can begin to interpret these signals and respond in ways that bring you relief and comfort. Let's decipher this new language together, starting with identifying triggers, exploring cooling techniques, and considering how your choice of clothing can make a big difference.

Identifying Triggers

Hot flashes are sudden sensations of warmth, often most intense over the face, neck, and chest, with accompanying reddening of the skin, as if you're blushing. Sweating, especially in the upper body, often follows this rush of heat. The exact cause of hot flashes isn't fully understood, but they're likely related to the hormonal changes that occur during menopause.

Triggers can be seen as the ignition for these hot flashes—the spark that sets off the heat wave. Identifying your unique triggers is like learning the alphabet of this new body language. Common triggers include spicy foods, caffeine, alcohol, stress, tight clothing, heat, and cigarette smoke.

Keeping a journal can be a great way to pinpoint your triggers. When a hot flash strikes, note what you were doing, eating, or feeling at the time. Over time, you may start to see patterns emerge, offering valuable insight into your personal triggers.

Cooling Techniques

Once you've identified potential triggers, the next step is to find effective ways to cool down when a hot flash strikes. Think of these as your body's 'cooling-off' phases in response to the heated conversation of hot flashes.

One simple technique is to practice deep, slow breathing as soon as a hot flash begins. This technique, known as paced respiration, can help to reduce the intensity of hot flashes. Another strategy is to use a handheld fan or a cold pack on your neck or face during a hot flash.

Remember to stay hydrated by drinking cool water throughout the day. Also, a spray bottle filled with cool water can provide instant relief when a hot flash strikes. If you're at home when a hot flash begins, try to move to a cooler part of your house or open a window to let in some fresh air.

Dressing for Comfort

Your wardrobe can play a big role in managing hot flashes. Dressing for comfort is like choosing the proper attire for a weather forecast that includes sporadic heatwaves.

Dress in layers so that you can remove clothing when you feel a hot flash coming on. Choose clothes made from natural fibers, like cotton, which allow your skin to breathe. Avoid synthetic fabrics, like polyester, which can trap heat.

Wearing a cotton nightgown or pajamas can also help manage night sweats, ensuring your sleep isn't disrupted by sudden waves of heat. Additionally, consider keeping extra layers nearby when you sleep so you can add or remove them as needed.

Hot flashes and night sweats may seem like an odd language for your body to speak. However, you can effectively decode this language by identifying triggers, practicing cooling techniques, and dressing for comfort. In doing so, you'll gain a sense of control over your experience with menopause, turning these seemingly random bursts of heat into a dialogue you can navigate and understand.

Remember that the language of menopause, much like any foreign language, takes time to learn. Be patient with yourself, keep an open mind, and know that with each hot flash decoded, you're becoming more fluent in understanding your body's needs during this transition.

WEIGHT GAIN AND METABOLISM: THE DIET DILEMMA

Navigating the landscape of menopause often feels like a tightrope walk—a delicate balancing act. One of the most challenging aspects of this balance is managing weight gain and changes to your metabolism. It's like waking up one day to find your favorite jeans no longer fit or that the number on the scale has crept up seemingly overnight.

This weight gain, often concentrated around the abdomen, is a common symptom of menopause, and it's linked to fluctuating hormone levels and changes in metabolism.

Unraveling the connection between weight gain and menopause can feel like solving a complex puzzle. Still, understanding paired with strategic lifestyle adjustments can help you solve this puzzle and regain control over your body's evolving rhythm. Let's explore how nutrient-dense foods, portion control, and hydration can help you balance your metabolism and manage weight gain during menopause.

Nutrient-Dense Foods

Like a trusted compass guiding you through an unknown terrain, nutrient-dense foods can steer you towards healthier eating habits during the life stage of menopause. Nutrient-dense foods are those that pack a lot of beneficial nutrients into relatively few calories. They're like the superheroes of your diet, offering powerful nutritional benefits without the excess calories that can lead to weight gain.

Incorporating these nutrient powerhouses into your diet can help balance your metabolism and manage weight gain. These include colorful fruits and vegetables, lean proteins, whole grains, and healthy fats. Each of these foods brings something unique to the table.

Fruits and vegetables are rich in vitamins and minerals, offering antioxidants that promote overall health. Lean proteins, such as chicken, fish, eggs, and legumes, keep you feeling full and satisfied, preventing you from overeating. Whole grains offer fiber, aiding digestion and helping to control blood sugar levels. Healthy fats, which can be found in avocados, nuts, seeds, and fatty fish, support brain health and help your body absorb nutrients.

Portion Control

If nutrient-dense foods act as the compass guiding your menopause diet, portion control serves as the map outlining your journey. Portion control involves understanding how much food your body needs and adjusting your portions accordingly. Often, we eat with our eyes, based on visual cues, not realizing that our plates often hold more food than our bodies need.

Mastering portion control is like learning to read a new map. You need to understand the landmarks, the signs, and the distances between them. In terms of portion control, this translates to understanding what a portion size should look like for different types of food and practicing measuring or estimating these portions accurately.

For instance, a portion of lean protein should be about the size and thickness of your palm. Cooked grains or starchy vegetables should fit in your cupped hand, while a portion of raw, leafy vegetables should fit in two hands cupped together. Practicing portion control can help you avoid consuming excess calories, supporting weight management during menopause.

Hydration

Staying hydrated is another crucial element of managing weight gain and metabolism changes during menopause. Think of it like ensuring your vehicle has enough fuel for a journey ahead. Water is vital in many bodily functions, including digestion and nutrient absorption.

Maintaining hydration can also help regulate feelings of hunger. Thirst can often be mistaken for hunger, leading to unnecessary snacking. By staying hydrated, you can mitigate these false hunger signals. Aim for at least eight glasses of water daily, more if you're physically active. Herbal teas and fruit-infused waters can also contribute to your hydration, providing a flavorful twist to your daily hydration routine.

Weight gain and changes in metabolism can pose challenges during menopause. Yet, through understanding these changes and implementing strategic lifestyle adjustments, you can navigate this aspect of menopause with confidence. By incorporating nutrient-dense foods into your diet, practicing portion control, and prioritizing hydration, you can support your body's evolving rhythm, manage weight gain, and maintain your overall health and well-being during menopause.

MOOD SWINGS AND BRAIN FOG: THE EMOTIONAL DANCE

Menopause can sometimes feel like an unexpected dance partner, leading you into a whirl of emotions that can be both confusing and overwhelming. The fluctuating hormone levels can trigger mood swings and brain fog, creating the sensation of being caught in a tango that you didn't sign up for. However, with the right techniques, you can turn this tango into a waltz, gracefully navigating the emotional dance of menopause.

Navigating Cognitive Changes

At times, the journey through menopause might resemble a frenzied cha-cha, leaving you feeling strained and submerged. Yet, embracing certain strategies can help dial down the tempo, allowing you to traverse this life stage with greater poise and mastery.

The hormonal shifts of menopause can manifest in a myriad of ways, such as forgetfulness, sleep disturbances, and hot flashes. Ovarian health is intertwined with the function of the brain. As estrogen levels dip, there are alterations in the form, quantity, and interactions among the nerve cells.

Depending on where you are in the menopause journey, alterations in brain structure, neural connections, and energy metabolism are likely. Areas responsible for higher cognitive functions are particularly susceptible to changes. In the post-menopausal phase, one of the earliest shifts is a dip in glucose levels, which can result in reduced brain activity, given that glucose is crucial for optimal brain function.

This decline in glucose is linked to diminished estrogen levels. There might also be a reduction in grey matter due to hormone replacement. However, these shifts can vary significantly among women. Those in good health might experience only minor cognitive shifts compared to those with pre-existing health issues.

In essence, regardless of your health status, you might notice changes such as memory lapses, challenges with short-term recall and focus, a sense of mental haze, mood fluctuations, irritability, heightened risk of depression, and more. You might find that processing information takes a bit longer than it did during your reproductive years.

Much like a dancer adapting to the rhythm and nuances of a new routine, embracing useful strategies can help you navigate these changes with elegance and assurance. In the following sections, we'll explore each of these experiences and discover ways to waltz through them gracefully.

Stress Management Techniques

The dance of menopause can sometimes feel like a fast-paced salsa, leaving you feeling stressed and overwhelmed. However, adopting stress management techniques can help slow the music, allowing you to move with more ease and control.

One such technique is mindfulness, a practice of being fully present and engaged in the current moment. It's like finding a quiet corner in a bustling dance hall, a space where you can breathe, focus, and regain your footing. Mindfulness can be practiced anytime, anywhere—while eating, walking, or even during a quiet moment in your day.

Another effective stress management technique is progressive muscle relaxation, which is a method that involves tensing and then releasing each muscle group in your body. It's similar to a dancer stretching before a performance, releasing tension and preparing the body for the dance ahead.

Regular physical activity can also be a powerful stress buster. Whether it's a brisk walk, a yoga class, or a dance session in your living room—moving your body can trigger the release of endorphins, the body's natural stress relievers. Physical activity can lead to a feeling akin to the euphoria a dancer experiences after a successful performance—a natural high that lifts your mood and reduces stress.

Brain-Boosting Activities

Just as a dancer needs to remember complex choreography, maintaining mental sharpness during menopause can be a valuable part of your emotional well-being. Brain fog, characterized by periods of forgetfulness or lack of mental clarity, is a common symptom of menopause.

Engaging in brain-boosting activities can help clear the fog and sharpen your mental acuity. Think of these activities as a workout for your brain, strengthening your cognitive abilities like physical exercise strengthens your muscles.

Reading, solving puzzles, learning a new skill, or even playing memory-boosting games can stimulate your brain, keeping it active and agile. Like a dancer constantly learning new steps and routines, it's essential to keep the mind engaged and sharp.

Social engagement can also be a powerful brain booster. Participating in social activities or spending time with friends and family can stimulate your mind, reduce stress, and promote your overall well-being. Like a dancer feeding off the energy of the crowd, socializing will allow you to draw strength and motivation from connecting.

Emotional Support Networks

Navigating the emotional dance of menopause can sometimes feel like a solo performance, leaving you feeling isolated and misunderstood. However, you're not alone on this dance floor. Building an emotional support network can provide the companionship, understanding, and guidance you need during this transition.

This network can be composed of friends, family, health-care providers, or even support groups comprised of women going through a similar experience. It's like having a team of choreographers, dancers, and cheer-leaders all supporting you through your performance.

A support network can provide a safe space to express your feelings, share experiences, and seek advice. It's like a dancer's dressing room—a sanctuary where fears, doubts, and triumphs can be shared openly and without judgment.

Remember, the emotional dance of menopause is not one you have to perform alone. With stress management techniques, brain-boosting activities, and an emotional support network, you can navigate this dance with grace, confidence, and a strong sense of self.

SLEEP DISRUPTIONS: STRATEGIES FOR RESTFUL NIGHTS

Entering the realm of menopause can often feel like stepping onto a bustling dance floor, where the rhythm is ever-changing, and the music never seems to stop. Sleep disruptions, one of the most common complaints during menopause, can add to this feeling of constant movement, making it difficult to find moments of rest and rejuvenation. However, with a few strategic adjustments, you can slow the music and find your rhythm amid the hustle and bustle of menopause.

Sleep Hygiene Practices

Think of sleep hygiene as the choreography of your nightly routine. It's a series of steps designed to guide you towards restful and rejuvenating sleep. Good sleep hygiene involves:

- Maintaining a consistent sleep schedule.
- Creating a relaxing pre-sleep routine.
- Making your sleep environment as comfortable as possible.

Sticking to a consistent sleep schedule, where you go to bed and wake up at the same time every day, can help regulate your body's internal clock. Just as a dancer relies on the rhythm of the music, your body thrives on routine. By setting and maintaining a sleep schedule, you're providing a steady rhythm for your body to follow.

Creating a relaxing pre-sleep routine can signal to your body that it's time to wind down and prepare for sleep. This might involve activities like reading a book, taking a warm bath, or practicing gentle yoga. Like a dancer warming up before a performance, you are preparing the body for the routine ahead.

Relaxation Techniques

Relaxation techniques are like the slow, calming music that brings balance to a fast-paced dance playlist. These techniques can help reduce stress, promote relaxation, and prepare your body for sleep. Techniques like deep breathing, progressive muscle relaxation, or guided imagery can be particularly effective.

Deep breathing involves taking slow, deep breaths and focusing your attention on the sensation of the breath entering and leaving your body. It's like listening to the soft, steady rhythm of a slow dance song, bringing forth calm and focus.

Progressive muscle relaxation, on the other hand, involves tensing and then relaxing each muscle group in your body, starting from your toes and working your way up to your head. It's like a dancer methodically stretching each muscle, releasing tension and promoting relaxation.

Guided imagery involves visualizing a peaceful scene or situation. Like a dancer closing their eyes and imagining the dance floor, you're allowing your mind to create a sense of calm and peace.

Bedroom Environment Adjustments

Adjusting your bedroom environment can significantly impact the quality of your sleep. Think of it like setting the stage for a dance performance. Just as the lighting, sound, and layout of a stage can influence a dancer's performance, the conditions in your bedroom can impact your sleep.

Keeping your bedroom cool, dark, and quiet can create optimal conditions for sleep. Consider using earplugs or a white noise machine to block out disruptive noises, and use blackout curtains or an eye mask to keep your room dark. A cool room temperature, around 60-67 degrees Fahrenheit, is typically ideal for sleeping.

Your choice of bedding can also influence your sleep. Choose comfortable, breathable sheets and blankets, and find a pillow that supports your neck and head. Consider a mattress that provides the right amount of support and comfort.

Sleep disruptions may be a common part of the menopause experience, but they don't have to take center stage. With good sleep hygiene, relaxation techniques, and a few adjustments to your bedroom environment, you can create a sleep routine that supports restful nights and energized days. So, take a deep breath, find your rhythm, and dance into the restful sleep you deserve.

And as we bring the curtain down on this chapter, let's take the knowledge we've acquired into the next phase of our exploration. Are you ready? Great. Let's move to the beat of newfound understanding and continue our dance through the world of menopause. Don't worry; you're doing great. After all, every skilled dancer was once a beginner. Let's keep learning, growing, and dancing together.

Checklist: Daily Symptom Tracker

Monitor your symptoms daily to help identify patterns and triggers.

Please check the symptoms you experienced today:

- Hot flashes
- Night sweats
- Sleep disturbances
- Weight gain or increased appetite
- Mood swings or irritability
- Brain fog or memory issues
- Fatigue or low-energy
- Vaginal dryness or discomfort
- Decrease in libido
- Joint or muscle pain

Interactive Element: Symptom Intensity Rating Scale

Understanding the intensity of your symptoms can help when discussing them with your healthcare provider.

For each symptom you experienced today, rate its intensity on a scale of 1 to 10 (1 being very mild and 10 being very severe):

Hot flashes: __/10

Night sweats: __/10

Sleep disturbances: __/10

Weight gain or increased appetite: __/10

Mood swings or irritability: __/10

Brain fog or memory issues: __/10

Fatigue or low energy: __/10

Vaginal dryness or discomfort: __/10

Decrease in libido: __/10

Joint or muscle pain: __/10

To-Do: Start a Symptom Journal

Keeping a journal focused on your menopause symptoms can be a helpful tool in understanding your body's changes and discussing them with your healthcare provider.

- Get a dedicated notebook or digital app: This will be your symptom journal. Choose whatever method feels most comfortable and accessible to you.
- Date each entry: This will help you track your symptoms over time and identify any patterns.
- Note the time of day for each symptom: Some symptoms might be related to specific times of the day.
- Detail the symptom: Describe what you felt, how long it lasted, and any potential triggers (e.g., spicy food leading to a hot flash).

- Include your emotional state: Your emotional well-being can impact and be impacted by your symptoms.
- Review weekly: At the end of each week, take a moment to review your entries. This can help you identify any patterns or triggers, which will be helpful when discussing your symptoms with a healthcare professional.

3

PHYSICAL HEALTH IMPLICATIONS

BONE HEALTH: FORTIFYING YOUR FRAME

Menopause is a natural stage in a woman's life, signifying the conclusion of her menstrual cycles. It marks a period of significant physiological changes, many of which carry far-reaching health implications. Among the most important considerations during and after this transition is bone health.

As we explore the vital aspect of postmenopausal well-being, it's imperative to approach the subject with sensitivity. After all, the body's metamorphosis is not just a series of clinical symptoms to be managed; it is a profoundly personal journey that touches the core of a woman's sense of self and vitality.

Understanding the Link Between Menopause and Bone Health

Bones are living tissue, continually undergoing a process of breakdown and rebuilding. Estrogen, a hormone that diminishes during menopause, is crucial in maintaining bone density. The decrease in estrogen levels can result in an acceleration of bone loss, heightening the risk for osteoporosis—a condition where bones become fragile and more susceptible to fractures.

For many women, the first realization of changes in bone density occurs during an unexpected fracture or a routine bone density scan. While this moment can be challenging, knowledge and preparation can be empowering allies in navigating this new phase.

Early Prevention and Detection

Empowerment begins with prevention and early detection. Bone density peaks in your 20s and starts declining with age. By the time you reach menopause, this decline accelerates, underscoring the importance of adopting bone-strengthening habits early. These include:

- Calcium and Vitamin D Intake: Ensuring a diet rich in calcium and vitamin D is crucial for bone health. Leafy greens, dairy products, and fortified foods, along with sunlight exposure and supplements, if needed, can contribute to this effort.

- Regular Exercise: Engaging in weight-bearing and muscle-strengthening exercises such as walking, jogging, or resistance training, can help slow down bone loss.
- Healthy Lifestyle Choices: Taking significant steps, such as quitting smoking and moderating alcohol consumption, is crucial, as both habits can accelerate bone loss.

Early detection through bone density tests allows you and your healthcare provider to formulate a plan to protect your bone health. These quick, painless tests provide a wealth of information about your bone health status.

Navigating Treatment Options

If osteoporosis becomes a concern, several treatments and medications are available to reduce bone loss and the risk of fractures. Hormone replacement therapy (HRT) has demonstrated efficacy in preventing bone loss and lowering fracture risk in postmenopausal women. However, its suitability varies due to potential risks and side effects.

Bisphosphonates, a commonly prescribed class of drugs, aim to prevent bone density loss, and newer medications with different mechanisms of action are also available. It's essential to discuss the risks and benefits of these treatments with your healthcare provider in order to make informed decisions that align with your personal health profile and preferences.

The Emotional Dimension of Bone Health

Beyond the physical aspect of bone health, the emotional dimension is equally vital. The realization that one's bones are becoming more fragile can sometimes bring about feelings of vulnerability. Support groups, counseling, and open conversations with loved ones can offer valuable emotional sustenance.

Remember, while menopause is a universal experience, each woman's journey is unique. Seeking community and shared experiences can provide strength, with encouragement and understanding from peers serving as a balm during times of uncertainty.

The transition to menopause is a complex period where bone health warrants particular attention. You can protect your bones with mindful lifestyle choices, vigilant monitoring, and the appropriate use of medical therapies when necessary. Navigating this natural evolution of life requires patience, care, and, above all, compassion for oneself. As you traverse this journey, remember that your well-being is holistic, encompassing the body, mind, and spirit.

HEART HEALTH: THE HEART'S JOURNEY THROUGH MENOPAUSE

The years surrounding menopause constitute a pivotal period for a woman's heart health. As estrogen levels decline, the protective effects of this hormone on the circulatory system diminish, rendering women more vulnerable to cardiovascular disease. A nuanced understanding of the changes occurring during this phase is vital to navigating heart health with wisdom and care.

The Menopause Transition and the Heart

Menopause isn't solely a reproductive milestone; it marks a significant shift in a woman's cardiovascular risk profile. Before menopause, women typically enjoy a lower risk of heart disease compared to men, partly due to estrogen's beneficial influence on cholesterol levels and blood vessel flexibility. As menopause approaches, the decrease in estrogen disrupts this advantage, coinciding with an uptick in heart-related concerns.

One of the most insidious threats is the gradual buildup of plaque in the arteries, a condition known as atherosclerosis. This buildup can lead to heart attacks and strokes if not managed effectively. Changes in cholesterol levels, marked by an increase in the "bad" LDL cholesterol and a decrease in the "good" HDL cholesterol, further contribute to this risk. Additionally, blood pressure often rises during menopause, imposing additional strain on the heart and vascular system.

Symptom Recognition and Misconceptions

Women may experience symptoms of heart disease differently than men. It is not uncommon for women to report fatigue, shortness of breath, and a feeling of indigestion rather than the classic chest pain. These subtler signs can be misleading, emphasizing the importance of awareness and education about the manifestation of heart disease in women.

During menopause, a period already marked by significant bodily changes, distinguishing between typical menopausal symptoms and potential signs of more serious concerns can be challenging. Hot flashes, for instance, have been associated with cardiovascular changes. While they are a normal part of menopause, they should not be dismissed if they coincide with other symptoms and indications of heart distress.

Lifestyle Strategies for Heart Health

The heart, however, is a responsive organ, and lifestyle adjustments can significantly impact its well-being. Here are several empowering steps women can take:

- Diet: A heart-healthy diet rich in fruits, vegetables, lean proteins, and whole grains while minimizing saturated fats, cholesterol, and sodium can help manage cholesterol levels and blood pressure.

- Exercise: Regular physical activity contributes to maintaining a healthy weight, lowering blood pressure, improving cholesterol levels, and enhancing overall heart function. Aim for at least 150 minutes of moderate-intensity exercise per week.
- Stress Management: Menopause, with its hormonal fluctuations and life changes, can be a stressful period in a woman's life. Chronic stress can negatively affect heart health, making it beneficial to incorporate stress-reduction techniques such as meditation, deep breathing exercises, or yoga.
- Smoking Cessation: Quitting smoking is a pivotal decision for heart health, considering that smoking is a major risk factor for heart disease.
- Moderate Alcohol Intake: Excessive alcohol consumption can increase blood pressure and contribute to extra calorie intake, potentially leading to weight gain. Moderation is key.

Medical Interventions and Support

Beyond lifestyle adjustments, medical interventions can also play a role in heart health. Blood pressure medications, cholesterol-lowering drugs, and other treatments may be necessary to manage risk factors effectively.

Hormone Replacement Therapy (HRT) has been the subject of much debate. While it may alleviate some menopausal symptoms, it is not universally recommended for heart disease prevention. HRT should be tailored to individual cases and discussed with a healthcare provider.

Regular check-ups are vital to ensure your heart health is on the right track. Women should feel empowered to openly discuss their concerns, especially regarding how menopause may be impacting their hearts, with their healthcare providers.

Embracing the Journey

While menopause introduces new challenges for heart health, it also presents an opportunity to adopt healthier habits and forge a path toward overall well-being. Understanding the heart's needs during this transition can empower women to make informed choices that enhance their quality of life during menopause and beyond. It's not just about extending years to life but also about adding life to those years by nurturing one of the most vital organs in our body—the heart.

BREAST HEALTH: UNDERSTANDING CHANGES

As women approach and transition through menopause, the topic of breast health assumes a prominent place in the tapestry of their overall well-being. This period of change, while a natural stage in the rhythm of life, brings a suite of considerations that demand our understanding and attention.

Understanding Changes in Breast Tissue

During menopause, the body undergoes significant hormonal fluctuations, which can have a tangible impact on breast tissue. Declining levels of estrogen and progesterone may lead to changes that many women experience as tenderness, swelling, or even discomfort. The once dense and glandular tissue may become more fatty and less firm—a transformation that is as much a part of the natural aging process as the graying of hair or the deepening of laugh lines.

While often benign, these changes require a gentle approach grounded in empathy and awareness. It's a time when listening to the body's signals becomes even more critical. Regular self-examinations become not just a practice in health maintenance but also an act of self-care—a way for women to remain connected to their bodies and attuned to any changes that may arise.

Navigating Breast Health Concerns

It is paramount during this stage to adhere to a routine of regular clinical breast exams and mammograms as recommended by healthcare professionals. The risk of breast cancer increases with age, and menopause presents a critical timeframe for vigilant screening. Empowerment comes from understanding risk factors, recognizing symptoms, and actively participating in health strategies, all of which can significantly affect outcomes.

However, beyond the clinical dimension, the emotional landscape of breast health can be complex. The intersection of identity, femininity, and the physical self may evoke feelings of vulnerability. Empathy should be the foundation of conversations and consultations, emphasizing respect for the individual and acknowledging the emotional aspects of physical health.

Lifestyle Considerations for Breast Health

Lifestyle choices play a substantial role in supporting breast health during menopause. A well-balanced diet rich in antioxidants and low in saturated fats contributes to overall well-being and may potentially reduce cancer risk. Physical activity also serves as a stronghold of health, helping regulate hormones, supporting weight management, and enhancing mood.

Factors like alcohol consumption and smoking can compromise breast health, making it advisable to moderate intake or abstain. Additionally, managing stress, which is often overlooked, is integral. Mindfulness practices, yoga, or simple daily relaxation techniques can mitigate the adverse effects of stress on the body's systems.

Support and Resources

It's important to remember that no woman is alone on this journey. Support groups, whether in-person or online communities, can provide camaraderie and understanding. Healthcare providers serve as knowledgeable guides, while friends and family offer a network of care and support.

In this chapter of life, a woman's relationship with her body may change, but it remains a source of strength and resilience. The commitment to breast health is a testament to the respect for the life lived and the years ahead— each check-up, each balanced meal, and each moment of rest is a step toward nurturing the self.

As women navigate the currents of menopause, breast health serves as a beacon, underscoring the importance of care and vigilance. With an empathetic approach, informed understanding, and supportive care, the journey through menopause can be navigated with grace and confidence, ensuring that breast health remains a priority on the path to enduring wellness.

HEALING APPROACHES: TAILORING YOUR THERAPEUTIC PATHWAY

As we conclude our exploration of bone, heart, and breast health in the context of menopause, it is clear that the transition through this natural phase of life demands a holistic approach to health and well-being. The following treatments and remedies are woven with the threads of compassion and understanding, acknowledging the unique journey each woman experiences.

Embracing a Multifaceted Approach

Bone Health: The demineralization of bones post-menopause is a silent process that often escapes notice until a fracture occurs. Addressing this involves foundational calcium and vitamin D supplementation, which forms just one part of the larger tapestry. Weight-bearing exercises, such as walking or lightweight training, fortify bone density and enhance muscle strength, providing a protective embrace for the skeletal system. Additionally, healthcare providers may recommend medications like bisphosphonates or hormone replacement therapy (HRT) for those at high risk of osteoporosis. Each treatment plan should be as unique as the individual, taking into account personal health history and risk factors.

Heart Health: The heart, that tireless engine, faces new challenges as estrogen levels diminish. Here, the remedy lies in nurturing the heart through diet and lifestyle. A diet rich in omega-3 fatty acids, fiber, and antioxidants supports heart function, while minimizing saturated fats and processed sugars helps maintain arterial health. Exercise becomes an ally, strengthening the heart and improving circulation. When lifestyle changes alone are insufficient, a healthcare professional may prescribe statins or blood pressure medications. Above all, regular check-ups enable early detection and management of potential heart health issues.

Breast Health: Vigilance in breast health is vital during and after menopause. Regular self-examinations and mammograms are of utmost importance in the early detection of breast anomalies. For those experiencing increased risk or discomfort, treatments may include selective estrogen receptor modulators (SERMs) or aromatase inhibitors under strict medical guidance. Including foods high in antioxidants and fiber, alongside a reduction in alcohol consumption, has been shown to support breast health. In all cases, continued dialogue with healthcare professionals ensures a treatment plan that is not only preventative but personalized.

Integrative Remedies

Menopause is not a disease but a natural transition, and the remedies we seek should not just address the physical symptoms but also honor the psychological and emotional changes that are occurring. Mind-body practices such as yoga and meditation can ease menopausal symptoms by reducing stress and promoting a sense of calm and balance. Support groups and therapy can also provide a space to share experiences and strategies, creating a community of support and understanding.

For holistic well-being, consider:

- Phytoestrogens: Found in soy, flaxseed, and other plant-based foods, these natural compounds can mimic the effects of estrogen in the body, potentially easing menopausal symptoms.

- Herbal Supplements: Herbs such as black cohosh, red clover, and evening primrose oil have traditionally been used for menopause symptom relief, though one should consult with a healthcare provider before starting any new supplement.
- Acupuncture: This traditional Chinese medicine practice has shown some efficacy in managing hot flashes and menopausal discomfort.

Personalized Care

Ultimately, the most effective treatment and remedy plan is one that is tailored to the individual. Collaborating closely with healthcare providers to monitor the impact of menopause on bone, heart, and breast health is crucial, allowing for adjustments to treatments as necessary. Regular screenings, informed lifestyle choices, and a proactive approach to symptom management can lead to a smoother transition through menopause and beyond.

As you navigate these changes, let compassion and self-care serve as your guiding principles. Celebrate your body's resilience, seek support when needed, and embrace this phase of life with knowledge and grace. With the proper care, menopause can evolve into a time of renewal and empowerment.

Self-Assessment Quiz: Understanding Your Health Journey

Instructions: Answer each question to the best of your knowledge. Review your answers at the end of the quiz to see which areas you might need more information on or areas to focus on for your health.

Bone Health:

How often do you perform weight-bearing exercises (like walking, jogging, or dancing)?

a) Daily
b) 2-3 times a week
c) Rarely or never

Do you consume calcium-rich foods or supplements regularly?

a) Yes, daily
b) Occasionally
c) Rarely or never

Heart Health:

How often do you check your blood pressure and cholesterol levels?

a) Regularly (at least once a year)
b) Occasionally
c) I don't remember the last time

How effectively do you manage stress, which is a known risk factor for heart disease?

a) Very effectively - I regularly practice stress management techniques
b) Moderately - I occasionally engage in stress-reducing activities
c) Not effectively - I rarely manage stress or am unsure how to

Breast Health:

Do you perform regular self-examinations for breast health?

a) Yes, monthly
b) Occasionally
c) Rarely or never

Have you discussed breast health changes during menopause with your healthcare provider?

a) Yes
b) Planned but not yet
c) No

Scoring: For each 'a' answer give yourself 2 points, for 'b' 1 point, and for 'c' 0 points. A higher score indicates better awareness and proactive management of your health during menopause.

Personalized Health Plan Template: My Menopause Health Plan

Instructions: Fill out each section with your personal goals and action steps based on the chapter's content.

Bone Health Goals:

Goal (e.g., Increase bone density):

Action Steps (e.g., Schedule weight-bearing exercises three times a week, increase calcium intake):

Heart Health Goals:

Goal (e.g., Improve cardiovascular health):

Action Steps (e.g., Regular blood pressure and cholesterol checks, incorporating heart-healthy foods):

Breast Health Goals:

Goal (e.g., Monitor changes during menopause):

Action Steps (e.g., Monthly self-examinations, schedule a mammogram):

Notes: Add any additional notes, concerns, or questions to discuss with your healthcare provider.

Weekly Wellness Tracker: Menopause Wellness Weekly Tracker

Instructions: Use this tracker to monitor your daily activities and health observations. This can help you stay on track with your health goals and notice any changes.

Week of [Date Range]:

Bone Health:

Weight-bearing exercises completed:
Calcium intake (diet/supplements):

Heart Health:

Cardiovascular exercises:
Heart-healthy meals:

Breast Health:

Self-examination done (Yes/No):
Any changes or discomfort noticed:

Weekly Reflection: At the end of the week, reflect on your achievements and areas that need more attention. Use this template to continue weekly tracking in your journal.

4

HORMONE REPLACEMENT THERAPY: UNRAVELING THE ENIGMA

I magine standing at the entrance of a labyrinth, holding a golden key in your hand. You've heard tales of a treasure hidden deep within the maze—a treasure that can ease your menopausal symptoms and improve your quality of life. It's said that this key in your hand can unlock the path to that treasure. But you're hesitant. You've also heard tales of hidden traps and potential dangers that lurk within the labyrinth. This is the enigma of Hormone Replacement Therapy (HRT)—a potential panacea for menopausal symptoms, yet one that comes with its share of questions and concerns. Let's unlock the mysteries of HRT together, understanding the basics, exploring the different types, and examining the various delivery methods.

DECODING HRT: THE BASICS

Understanding Hormone Replacement Therapy

Hormone Replacement Therapy, often abbreviated as HRT, is a treatment used to supplement the body with either estrogen alone or a combination of estrogen and progesterone. Think of it like adjusting a thermostat in a room that's becoming too cold. Just as you'd turn up the thermostat to warm the room, HRT increases the levels of these hormones in your body, aiming to alleviate the symptoms caused by their decline during menopause.

HRT can be particularly effective in treating common menopausal symptoms such as hot flashes, night sweats, mood swings, and vaginal dryness. It's like having a secret weapon in your arsenal, one that can help you combat these challenges and improve your quality of life.

Types of HRT

Like a professional artist's toolkit, HRT comes in various forms, each designed to cater to different needs and circumstances. Primarily, there are three types of HRT: Estrogen-only HRT, Combined HRT, and Local Estrogen.

1. Estrogen-only HRT is typically prescribed for women who have undergone a hysterectomy. It contains only estrogen and can be effective in treating symptoms like hot flashes and vaginal dryness. Think of it like a solo

dancer, taking the stage alone but still able to deliver a captivating performance.

2. Combined HRT, as the name suggests, combines estrogen with progesterone or a synthetic variant known as progestin. This combination can be a powerful force in alleviating a range of menopausal symptoms. Think of them like a pair of expert dancers working together to deliver a flawless performance.

3. Local Estrogen treatment comes in forms such as creams, rings, or tablets that are applied directly to the vagina to alleviate symptoms like dryness or discomfort during intercourse. It's like having a dedicated spotlight on stage, focusing its beam on a specific area.

Delivery Methods

HRT offers various delivery methods, each with its unique attributes. It's like choosing the right mode of transportation for a journey; while the destination remains the same, the journey itself might look different.

1. Pills are the most common form of HRT. They're taken orally, usually once a day. It's like taking a bus on a regular route—a familiar and straightforward method.

2. Skin Patches or gels allow the hormones to be absorbed directly through your skin. They're applied once or twice a week, offering a convenient option that bypasses the digestive system. Think of it like a scenic bike ride, offering a unique path to the same destination.

3. Vaginal Rings, Tablets, or Creams provide localized estrogen therapy, targeting specific symptoms like vaginal dryness or discomfort. It's like rowing a boat across a lake, a more targeted approach to reaching a specific location.

Understanding the basics of HRT is like having a detailed map of the labyrinth. It empowers you to make informed decisions about your health and menopausal treatment. As we deepen our exploration of the world of HRT, remember that this key you hold, the golden key of knowledge, can unlock the path to improved well-being and quality of life during the life stage of menopause. It's your guide through the enigma of HRT, illuminating the path and helping you confidently navigate the labyrinth.

THE PROS AND CONS: MAKING AN INFORMED DECISION

Benefits of HRT

Picture yourself out on a sunny day, donning a pair of sunglasses. While the shades don't stop the sun from shining, they do make it easier for you to see and move around without squinting or discomfort. In many ways, Hormone Replacement Therapy (HRT) operates similarly. It doesn't stop menopause, but it can make navigating the transition much smoother.

One of the most significant benefits of HRT is its effectiveness in treating typical menopausal symptoms. Hot flashes and night sweats, which can be frequent and severe for some women, often respond well to HRT. This therapy can be like finding an oasis in a desert, offering much-needed relief from the unrelenting heat.

The therapy is also beneficial for tackling issues of vaginal discomfort. Dryness, itching, and discomfort during intercourse, which can sneak up during menopause, find their match with HRT. This therapy is much like a soothing balm applied to a skin irritation.

Furthermore, HRT has a protective effect on bone health. It reduces the risk of osteoporosis, a condition that weakens bones and makes them more susceptible to fractures. It's like a safety net, providing additional protection to your skeletal structure.

Potential Side Effects

While HRT has advantages, it's essential to be aware of the potential side effects, much like reading the fine print before signing an agreement. In the initial stages of the therapy, some women might experience bloating, breast tenderness, nausea, and mood swings. These side effects are usually temporary and tend to subside as your body adjusts to the therapy, similar to the initial discomfort one might experience when breaking in a new pair of shoes.

However, some side effects can be more serious. HRT can slightly increase the risk of certain conditions like blood clots, stroke, and specific types of cancer. Making the decision to use this therapy is a bit like navigating a path with potential pitfalls. Awareness of these risks can help you be vigilant and proactive in your health care.

Long-Term Implications

HRT is not just about immediate relief from menopausal symptoms; it's also about considering the long-term implications for your health and well-being. It's like planting a tree, where the consequences of your actions will only become apparent with time.

The decision to start, continue, or stop HRT is not a one-time choice. It's a decision that needs to be revisited and reviewed regularly with your healthcare provider. It's like tuning a musical instrument, requiring regular adjustments to maintain the perfect balance.

The duration of HRT can also have different implications. Short-term use of HRT, generally considered up to five years, has been associated with minimal risks. However, using HRT for a longer duration or starting the therapy after the age of 60 might increase the risk of side effects and complications.

Arriving at a well-informed decision about HRT involves a thoughtful assessment of its benefits compared to the potential side effects and the long-term implications. This process is like balancing on a seesaw, demanding careful consideration and regular adjustments. And while navigating this balancing act can seem daunting, remember you're not alone. Your healthcare provider is there to guide and support you, ensuring you possess all the necessary information to make the best decision for your health and well-being.

NATURAL ALTERNATIVES TO HRT: HERBAL REMEDIES AND MORE

When sailing through the waves of menopause, some women might find themselves casting around for an alternative anchor, one that is rooted in nature and offers a more holistic approach. Enter the world of herbal remedies, a natural alternative to HRT that can provide relief from menopausal symptoms. Let's explore some of these natural allies, including phytoestrogens, black cohosh, and St. John's Wort.

Phytoestrogens

Phytoestrogens, a natural compound found in certain plants, have a similar structure to the estrogen produced by our bodies. Think of them like doppelgangers, nature's look-alikes, capable of performing a similar role, albeit with less intensity.

Certain foods are rich in these compounds, including soy products, flaxseed, and whole grains. Consuming these foods is like adding logs to a dwindling fire, providing a gentle boost to your body's declining estrogen levels.

While phytoestrogens might not be as potent as the estrogen used in HRT, they can still help manage mild menopausal symptoms. However, it's important to note that the effectiveness of phytoestrogens can vary from person to person, much like different dancers responding to the same music in their unique ways.

Black Cohosh

Black Cohosh, a plant native to North America, has a long history of being used for medicinal purposes, particularly for women's health issues. Think of this plant as a seasoned performer, tried and tested over centuries and recognized for its potential benefits.

Supplements made from black cohosh root can effectively alleviate hot flashes and night sweats. It's like having a personal fan, offering relief from the heat waves of menopause. However, as with any herbal supplement, it's important to use black cohosh under the guidance of a healthcare provider.

St. John's Wort

St. John's Wort, a flowering plant, is often used as a natural remedy for depression. Picture it as a ray of sunshine, known for its bright yellow flowers and potential to lift spirits.

Research suggests that St. John's Wort might help improve mood swings associated with menopause, providing a natural mood booster. It's like having a peaceful melody playing in the background, adding a sense of calm and balance to your transition to the life stage of menopause.

However, it's important to be aware that St. John's Wort can interact with certain medications, including birth control pills and some types of HRT. Hence, it's especially important to consult your healthcare provider before starting this or any herbal supplement.

Navigating the waves of menopause can be challenging, but you're not alone in this voyage. Whether you choose the boat of HRT or the raft of herbal remedies, remember that your destination remains the same—a place of balance, wellness, and empowered living. And as you sail these waters, remember that every wave and every gust of wind is a part of the adventure, shaping you into a stronger, more resilient sailor.

HAVING THE HRT CONVERSATION: QUESTIONS FOR YOUR HEALTHCARE PROVIDER

Navigating the waters of menopause is like piloting a ship through unfamiliar territories. The guide to steering the ship in the right direction lies in the compass of knowledge and understanding. In this journey, one of the critical conversations is with your healthcare provider about Hormone Replacement Therapy (HRT). To assist you in this crucial conversation, let's consider three key areas: Assessing your health history, discussing your symptoms, and exploring your options.

Assessing Your Health History

Your historical and present health status serves as the initial focal point of this discussion, much like the starting point on a map. Sharing your detailed health history with your healthcare provider is pivotal in determining the suitability of HRT for you. This process is like providing the prelude to a play before the curtains open.

This conversation includes disclosing information about any chronic conditions you may have, such as heart disease or diabetes, and any medications or supplements you're currently taking. Even details about lifestyle habits, like smoking and alcohol consumption, can have significant implications. Think about including these details like the brushstrokes that complete the canvas of your health portrait.

Family medical history, especially of conditions like breast cancer, ovarian cancer, or heart disease, can also impact the decision about HRT. It's similar to understanding the subtle influences that shape an intricate piece of music.

Discussing Your Symptoms

The next step in your conversation is to openly discuss the symptoms you're experiencing. Be candid about the physical and emotional symptoms of menopause that you're dealing with, whether it's hot flashes, night sweats, mood swings, or sleep disturbances.

Consider the frequency, intensity, and impact of these symptoms on your daily life. Are they like occasional gusts of wind or more like a persistent storm? Providing a clear picture of your symptoms can help your healthcare provider better understand your experience of menopause and guide you through the possibilities of managing these symptoms, including the potential use of HRT.

Exploring Your Options

Now that your health history and symptoms are on the table, you can finally explore options. Like a crossroad on a trail, this is where you consider the different paths that lie ahead. Discuss HRT's potential benefits and risks in the context of your personal health profile with your healthcare provider.

Ask about the different types of HRT and delivery methods, and discuss how they might suit your needs. This conversation is like understanding the nuances of various dance forms before deciding which resonates with you the most.

Additionally, consider exploring the alternatives to HRT. Ask about lifestyle modifications, natural remedies, or non-hormonal medications that could help manage your symptoms. This is like exploring the different routes to a destination before choosing the path that suits you best.

Having an open, informed conversation with your healthcare provider is a valuable step in navigating the uncharted waters of menopause. It equips you with the information you need to make decisions that fit your body's unique rhythm. It's about understanding your past, acknowledging your present, and making the best choices for your future.

As you continue to sail through the sea of menopause, remember that this voyage is uniquely your own. Each wave you navigate and decision you make shapes your personal journey towards balance, wellness, and empowered living. As we close this chapter, let's look forward to the next leg of our exploration, armed with the knowledge we've gained and the wisdom we've gathered. You're the captain of your ship, and with every wave and every gust of wind, you're becoming a more skilled and resilient sailor. Let the adventure continue!

Checklist: Benefits and Side-effects of HRT

Understanding HRT's potential benefits and side effects can help you make an informed decision.

Benefits of HRT:

- Relief from hot flashes and night sweats
- Improved sleep
- Reduced vaginal dryness and discomfort
- Possible reduction in mood swings
- Potential protection against osteoporosis

Side-effects of HRT:

- Nausea
- Bloating or water retention
- Tender or swollen breasts
- Headaches or migraines
- Mood changes
- Potential increased risk of certain cancers (e.g., breast cancer)
- Increased risk of blood clots or stroke

Note: The benefits and risks of HRT can vary from person to person. Having an in-depth discussion with your healthcare provider about your situation is crucial.

Interactive Element: Pros and Cons of HRT

This template will help you list your personal pros and cons regarding HRT as you understand them.

Pros of HRT for Me:

Cons of HRT for Me:

This exercise is designed to help you reflect on your individual perspective regarding HRT. By clearly identifying your pros and cons, you can better communicate your thoughts and concerns with your healthcare provider.

To-Do: Book an Appointment

Discussing HRT with a healthcare professional can provide clarity and confidence in your decision-making process.

- Research and Identify: If you don't already have a healthcare provider specializing in menopause or HRT, research and find recommended doctors in your area.
- Prepare Questions: Write down any questions or concerns you have about HRT. Use the pros and cons list you created to guide your conversation.
- Schedule the Appointment: Don't delay; the sooner you have the conversation, the sooner you can make informed decisions about your health.
- Document the Discussion: During or after your appointment, note the recommendations, answers to your questions, and any additional information your provider communicated.

5

NUTRITION FOR THE MENOPAUSAL BODY

Imagine yourself standing in a boxing ring. You're donned in gloves and facing an opponent named "Weight Gain." This opponent is notorious for its sneak attacks during the menopause phase. But guess what? You are not defenseless. Your arsenal is filled with potent strategies, and your most powerful weapon is food. Yes, food! Not just any food, but foods rich in nutrients, low in empty calories, and tailored to support your body during menopause.

In this chapter, we will focus on how food can be your ally in this battle against weight gain. We'll explore how portion control, fiber-rich foods, lean proteins, and healthy fats can help you keep weight gain at bay, maintain your energy levels, and support your overall health during menopause. So, put on your gloves, step into the ring, and get ready to fight back with food!

THE WEIGHT GAIN WAR: FIGHTING BACK WITH FOOD

Portion Control

One of the most effective strategies in the fight against weight gain is practicing portion control. Understanding portion control is like knowing exactly how much fuel your car needs to run efficiently without overfilling the tank. Even if it's healthy food, overeating can lead to weight gain because any extra calories your body doesn't burn are stored as fat.

Practicing portion control is about understanding what a serving size looks like for different types of food and ensuring your meals and snacks align with these guidelines. For instance, a portion of meat or protein should be approximately the size of your palm, while a portion of carbohydrates should be around the size of your fist.

A practical tip for implementing portion control is simply using smaller plates and bowls for your meals. This can trick your brain into thinking you're eating more than you are. Another helpful guideline is to fill half your plate with vegetables, a quarter with lean protein, and the remaining quarter with whole grains.

High Fiber Foods

Including more high-fiber foods in your diet is another effective strategy to manage weight gain during menopause. Fiber adds bulk to your diet and helps you feel full longer, which can help prevent overeating. It's like having a sturdy anchor that keeps your ship steady amid the waves of hunger.

High-fiber foods include fruits, vegetables, whole grains, and legumes. Try adding some berries to your breakfast, choosing whole grain bread for your sandwiches, or adding beans to your salad.

Lean Proteins

Protein stands out as an important nutrient for weight management because it aids in the development and preservation of muscle mass. And the more muscle you have, the more calories your body burns, even during periods of rest. It's like having a super-efficient engine that burns fuel even when you're not driving.

Opting for lean proteins like chicken, fish, eggs, and legumes is particularly beneficial. These protein sources provide the necessary building blocks for your body without the extra fat and calories. Think of them as a team of builders working to construct and repair your body's structural components.

Healthy Fats

While it may seem counterintuitive, including healthy fats in your diet can help you manage weight gain during menopause. Healthy fats like those found in avocados, nuts, seeds, and fatty fish can induce a sense of fullness, preventing overeating. It's like having a sturdy wall that keeps hunger at bay.

However, it's important to remember that healthy fats are still high in calories, so moderation is key. A small handful of nuts, a quarter of an avocado, or a piece of fatty fish like salmon are all effective ways to incorporate healthy fats into your diet.

Navigating menopause is like sailing through a storm, and weight gain can be one of the biggest waves you'll face. But with portion control, high-fiber foods, lean proteins, and healthy fats, you'll have the strategies to navigate these waves successfully. Remember, you're the captain of your ship, and every choice you make shapes your voyage. Choose wisely, eat well, and you'll sail through the storm into calmer waters.

THE MENOPAUSE-FRIENDLY KITCHEN: STAPLE FOODS

Preparing a menopause-friendly kitchen is like stocking your toolbox with the right tools. The more variety you have, the better equipped you are for the job. Let's unfold the toolkit and get acquainted with the indispensable tools—whole grains, fresh fruits and vegetables, dairy or dairy alternatives, and nuts and seeds.

Whole Grains

Step into the world of whole grains—a delightful assortment of nourishing foods integral to a menopause-friendly diet. Think of them like the sturdy foundation of a house, providing a stable base for your dietary structure.

Whole grains, including brown rice, quinoa, oats, and whole wheat, are packed with fiber. This nutrient is precious to your body during menopause, as it can help to manage weight and keep your digestive system running smoothly. Think of whole grains like a skillful plumber, ensuring the pipes in your house are unclogged and functioning optimally.

Moreover, whole grains are an excellent source of B vitamins, which are crucial for energy production. They are like the solar panels on a house, harnessing energy to keep the lights on. Including a variety of whole grains in your diet ensures that you feel full after you eat and are energized throughout the day.

Fresh Fruits and Vegetables

Now, take a moment to appreciate the vibrant colors in your toolkit. These are the fresh fruits and vegetables that you're including in your diet. They are like the beautiful paint that enhances the beauty of your house. Consuming a variety of fruits and vegetables can add a burst of flavor, texture, and color to your meals, making them more enjoyable.

Including fruits and vegetables in your diet is about more than aesthetics. They are nutritional powerhouses, abundant in vitamins, minerals, and antioxidants that support overall health. They are like the electrical wires in your house, transmitting necessary power to every corner.

Whether it's the Vitamin C in oranges boosting your immune system, the potassium in bananas supporting heart health, or the beta carotene in carrots promoting eye health, every fruit and vegetable brings something unique to your plate.

Dairy or Dairy Alternatives

Next, let's explore the role of dairy or dairy alternatives in a menopause-friendly diet. Think of this food group like the insulation in your house, playing a crucial role that often goes unnoticed. Dairy products like milk, cheese, and yogurt are excellent sources of calcium. This mineral is essential for bone health, particularly important during menopause due to the increased risk of osteoporosis.

If you're lactose intolerant or follow a vegan diet, plenty of dairy alternatives are available. Almond milk, soy milk, and rice milk are all excellent options. These alternatives are like eco-friendly insulation materials, serving the same purpose but with a different composition.

Nuts and Seeds

Lastly, let's not forget the small but mighty tools you'll need in your menopause-friendly diet—nuts and seeds.

They are like the nails and screws in your toolkit, small but essential for the overall structure. Nuts and seeds are nutritional gems packed with healthy fats, fiber, and a variety of vitamins and minerals.

Almonds, for instance, are a good source of Vitamin E, an antioxidant that protects your cells from damage. Flaxseeds are rich in Omega-3 fatty acids, which are beneficial for heart health. Chia seeds are packed with fiber, keeping you satiated while also supporting digestive health. Making sure to include a variety of nuts and seeds in your diet can significantly enhance the nutritional quality of your meals.

As we continue to navigate the world of menopause, remember that your kitchen is your sanctuary, and food is your ally. With the right tools—whole grains, fresh fruits and vegetables, dairy or dairy alternatives, and nuts and seeds—you will be well-equipped to manage the dietary challenges of menopause. And remember, every meal is an opportunity to nourish your body, so make the most of it by choosing foods that support your health and well-being during this unique phase of life.

RECIPES FOR RELIEF: SIMPLE, TASTY, AND HORMONE-BALANCING

Nourishing your body during menopause is like composing a symphony. Understanding your body's unique rhythm and flow will better allow you to create a harmonious balance. As you orchestrate your meals, consider the following recipes. They are not only delightful to your taste buds but also crafted to provide the nutrients your body needs during menopause.

Quinoa Salad with Fresh Veggies

Quinoa, a protein-packed grain, is the perfect base for a nutritious and satisfying salad. Think of it like a blank canvas, ready to be adorned with colorful, crunchy, and fresh vegetables.

To prepare this salad, cook a cup of quinoa per the package instructions. While the quinoa is simmering, chop your favorite vegetables. You can use bell peppers, cucumbers, cherry tomatoes, and red onions for a burst of color and nutrients.

Once the quinoa is cooked and cooled, mix in the vegetables. Add a handful of chopped fresh herbs like parsley or mint for an extra pop of flavor. Dress the salad with a simple vinaigrette of olive oil, lemon juice, salt, and pepper. This easy-to-make salad is not only vibrant and tasty, but it is also packed with fiber, protein, and various vitamins and minerals.

Baked Salmon with Lemon and Dill

Salmon, a fatty fish rich in omega-3 fatty acids, is a fantastic choice for a menopause-friendly diet, providing heart-healthy fats and high-quality protein to your meals.

To prepare this dish, preheat your oven to 375°F (190°C). Place a salmon fillet on a piece of foil large enough to fold over and seal. Top the salmon with thin slices of lemon and fresh dill sprigs. For added flavor, sprinkle some salt and pepper and a drizzle of olive oil. Fold the foil over the salmon and bake for about 15-20 minutes or until the salmon is cooked to your liking. This heart-healthy, flavorful dish is a testament that nutritious food can also be delicious.

Greek Yogurt Parfait with Berries and Granola

Greek yogurt, a powerhouse of protein and calcium, pairs beautifully with antioxidant-rich berries and crunchy granola in this parfait recipe. It's a harmonious trio, each ingredient complementing the others.

Begin by choosing a low-sugar, high-protein Greek yogurt. Layer it with fresh or frozen berries—blueberries, strawberries, raspberries, or a combination of these choices. Top this with a sprinkle of granola for a satisfying crunch. For added sweetness, drizzle a spoonful of honey or a sprinkle of cinnamon on top. This parfait makes a delightful breakfast or snack, offering a balance of protein, fiber, and antioxidants.

Stir-fried tofu with Vegetables

Tofu, an excellent plant-based protein and calcium source, shines in this easy stir-fry recipe. It's like a versatile dancer, ready to take on any rhythm in any style.

Start by pressing the tofu to remove excess moisture. The next step is to cut it into cubes and marinate it in a mixture of soy sauce, sesame oil, and a touch of honey. While the tofu is marinating, chop a variety of vegetables. Bell peppers, broccoli, carrots, and snap peas work well.

Heat a bit of oil in a pan, add the tofu cubes, and stir-fry until golden brown. Remove the tofu from the pan, add a bit more oil, and stir-fry the vegetables until they're tender-crisp. Add the tofu back to the pan, stir everything together, and voila! You now have a nutrient-dense, flavorful meal that's high in protein and packed with vitamins and minerals.

Feeding your body during menopause is not just about ticking off nutritional checkboxes. It's about enjoying a variety of foods, savoring each bite, and tuning into your body's unique needs. With these recipes in your repertoire, you're well-equipped to create meals that are nourishing and balanced but also delightful and satisfying. Bon Appétit!

DIETARY DON'TS: FOODS TO AVOID DURING MENOPAUSE

Processed Foods

In the symphony of menopause nutrition, processed foods hit a discordant note. Think of them like an ill-fitted piece in a well-crafted jigsaw puzzle. These foods, often high in salt, unhealthy fats, and additives, can exacerbate menopausal symptoms and increase the risk of weight gain and heart disease.

Processed foods include fast foods, packaged snacks, canned foods with added salt, and ready-to-eat meals. They might be convenient but lack the nutritional value your body needs during menopause. Think of them like shortcuts on a map that lead to a dead end.

High-Sugar Foods

High-sugar foods during menopause are like a siren's song—alluring but detrimental to your health. They can cause your blood sugar to spike and crash, leading to mood swings, fatigue, and weight gain.

These foods include candy, baked goods, sugary drinks, and even certain types of cereal. They might taste delightful, but they offer little nutritional value. Eating these high-sugar foods is like listening to a captivating melody that leaves you with a ringing noise in your ears.

Caffeine

Caffeine during menopause might give you a quick energy boost, but it can also lead to sleep disturbances and an increased heart rate.

If hot flashes are a part of your menopause experience, you might find that caffeine triggers or exacerbates these episodes. After drinking caffeine, it's like the dance suddenly speeds up, leaving you feeling overheated and uncomfortable.

Caffeine is found not just in coffee but also in tea, chocolate, and many soft drinks. If you're sensitive to its effects, consider reducing your intake or switching to decaffeinated versions of your favorite beverages.

Alcohol

Alcohol during the stage of menopause could be compared to a mirage in a desert. It might seem like a way to relax and cool down, but too much can lead to sleep problems, mood swings, and an increased risk of osteoporosis.

Alcohol can also trigger hot flashes and contribute to weight gain. It's like a detour on a road trip; it might seem fun at first, but it takes you further away from your destination.

While an occasional glass of wine is unlikely to do much harm, regular or heavy drinking can have significant health implications. It's all about finding a balance that works for you, ensuring that your intake doesn't steer you off the path to wellness.

Navigating the dietary landscape during menopause is about making conscious choices. It's about knowing which foods to embrace and which to limit or avoid. While the road might seem challenging, remember that every step you take is shaping your health and wellness.

So, as you map out your menopause-friendly diet, remember to tune into your body's unique needs and rhythms. Let it guide you towards foods that nourish and sustain and away from those that don't serve your health and overall well-being.

In the next chapter, we will continue to explore ways to support your body during menopause, focusing on the role of exercise and energy management. So, keep your compass at hand as we continue to chart the course of your voyage through menopause.

Checklist: Menopause-Friendly Foods to Stock

Prioritize these nutritious and menopause-supportive foods in your kitchen for optimal health during this life stage.

Whole Grains:

- Quinoa
- Oats
- Brown rice
- Barley

Proteins:

- Lentils
- Chickpeas
- Tofu
- Salmon

- Chicken breast

Dairy or Dairy Alternatives:

- Greek yogurt (unsweetened)
- Almond milk
- Soy milk (fortified)

Fruits & Vegetables:

- Leafy greens (e.g., kale, spinach)
- Broccoli
- Blueberries
- Avocado
- Bananas

Nuts & Seeds:

- Flaxseeds
- Chia seeds
- Almonds
- Walnuts

Herbs & Spices:

- Turmeric
- Ginger
- Cinnamon
- Black Cohosh

Regularly consuming these foods can provide essential nutrients to help manage menopause symptoms and support your overall health.

Interactive Element: "What's On My Plate?" Visual Guide

Using a visual representation can help guide balanced meal choices that are supportive of menopausal health. The aim is to ensure each meal contains essential food groups for optimal nutrition during menopause.

Instructions:

- Draw a Plate: On a blank sheet of paper, draw a large circle to represent your plate.
- Section the Plate: Divide the plate into four sections.
- Fill in the Sections:

  - Section 1 (50% of the plate): Fill with Fruits and vegetables. Color it in green. Key items include leafy greens, broccoli, carrots, bell peppers, apples, and berries.
  - Section 2 (25% of the plate): Fill with Whole Grains. Color it in brown. Key items include quinoa, brown rice, oats, and whole wheat pasta.
  - Section 3 (15% of the plate): Fill with Proteins. Color it in pink/red or beige for plant-based. Key items include chicken, fish, tofu, beans, and lentils.

- Section 4 (10% of the plate): Fill with Dairy or Dairy-Alternatives. Color it in blue or purple for alternatives. Key items include yogurt, milk, almond milk, and soy milk.
- Add small circles on the side for nuts and seeds, herbs, and spices. These represent added fats and flavors.

- Reflect on Your Meals: For a few days, at each meal, think about this plate. How closely does your actual meal resemble this balanced plate? What can you add or adjust to better align it with your goals?

This visual guide serves as a hands-on, tangible tool that readers can refer to when planning and assessing their meals, helping to ensure that they're nourishing their bodies appropriately during menopause.

To-Do: Clean Out Pantry of Dietary Don'ts

Making space for nutritious foods begins by clearing out items that aren't supportive of menopausal health.

- Read Labels: Look for hidden sugars, unhealthy fats, and high sodium content in the items in your pantry.
- Dispose of Old Items: Any expired or soon-to-expire foods that aren't menopause-friendly should be discarded.

- Limit Processed Foods: Foods that contain a long list of unrecognizable ingredients are probably not the best choice for your overall well-being. Consider reducing or eliminating these foods.
- Avoid Trigger Foods: If certain foods seem to exacerbate your menopause symptoms, it might be a good time to reduce or eliminate them.
- Restock with Care: After clearing out foods that aren't supportive of your menopausal health, make a list and shop for menopause-friendly foods. Use the checklist provided as a starting point.

SHARE YOUR INSIGHT, SHARE THE LIGHT!

A LITTLE KINDNESS GOES A LONG WAY.

"True generosity is giving without expecting applause or return—it's the silent applause of the heart."

— MOTHER TERESA

Hey there, wonderful reader! It's like we've been on an epic adventure together, exploring the twists and turns of menopause, right? And what an adventure it's been! Now, I've got a small favor to ask you...

Would you be the guiding star for someone just starting their journey?

Who is this person, you wonder? They're a bit like you before you had this book in your hands. They are eager to learn, yearning to make their way through the menopause maze, and looking for that light to help them navigate.

Our big dream is to make the wisdom of 'The Simple Menopause Manual' a lantern for everyone walking this path—everything I do springs from this dream. But to make it a reality, I need to reach...well, everyone.

This is your moment to shine! Many folks will select a book based on what others say about it (yes, the reviews!). So, here's my heartfelt request on behalf of a fellow navigator you've never met:

Please light their way by leaving a review for this book.

Your words are like a torch—costing you nothing but a minute of your time that can lead another person to clarity and confidence. Your review could be the beacon that helps:

...another person to breeze through their day without hot flashes.

...someone to feel strong and fit instead of worrying about weight.

...a friend to step off the wild hormone rollercoaster.

...a neighbor to embrace this change with joy rather than fear.

...another incredible woman to find her way to the other side.

To share that spark of joy and really make a difference, all it takes is a moment to leave a review.

Simply scan the QR code below to leave your review:

Or you go to the link below to leave your review:
http://tinyurl.com/2p864c2z

If the thought of helping someone out there makes your heart happy, then you're definitely my hero. Welcome to the club of light-sharers!

I can't wait to help you discover even more secrets to make your journey through menopause a joyful breeze. You're going to love the tips and tricks waiting for you in the next chapters.

Thank you from the deepest part of my heart. And now, let's dive back into our adventure!

Your biggest cheerleader,

Max Hampton

P.S. Did you know? When you share something valuable, you become someone's hero. And if you think this book could be their superhero cape, why not pass it on?

6

EXERCISE AND ENERGY: YOUR MENOPAUSE FITNESS GUIDE

P icture yourself on a dance floor, with the music pulsating through the speakers and the rhythm inviting you to move. The beat is catchy, and the melody is irresistible. You feel an urge to sway, tap your foot, and let your body respond to the music. This is the power of movement—the magic of exercise. During menopause, your body is like a dancer, responding to the rhythm of hormonal changes. In this dance, exercise becomes your choreography—a series of moves designed to support your body, balance your hormones, and enhance your well-being.

In the face of menopausal symptoms like hot flashes, mood swings, and weight gain, exercise can be a powerful ally. It's like a trusty sidekick in a superhero comic book, always ready to lend a hand in the battle against villainous symptoms. Regular physical activity can help regulate your hormones, manage your weight, boost your mood, and improve your overall health. It's the secret ingredient in your menopause survival kit, the golden thread intricately woven through the tapestry of your body's wellness.

THE BEST WORKOUT FOR YOUR HORMONES: A GUIDE TO MENOPAUSE-FRIENDLY EXERCISE

Low-Impact Cardio

Engaging in low-impact cardio exercises is like taking your body on a gentle hike. The terrain is smooth, and the pace is moderate, yet the benefits are significant. Activities like brisk walking, cycling, or swimming are easy on your joints while providing an excellent cardiovascular workout.

Think of low-impact cardio like walking through a garden. You're admiring the flowers and soaking in the sunshine. You're moving at your own pace, enjoying the journey, and your heart is still getting a good workout.

Strength Training

Strength training, on the other hand, is like lifting heavy boxes when you're reorganizing your house. It requires effort and can be challenging, but it makes you stronger and more resilient.

Whether lifting weights, using resistance bands, or doing exercises that use your body weight, like squats or push-ups, this training can help build muscle mass, boost your metabolism, and improve bone health. It's like building a solid foundation for your house, ensuring it is strong enough to withstand any storm.

Flexibility and Balance Exercises

Flexibility and balance exercises are essential in a well-rounded fitness routine, like fine-tuning a musical instrument. While not as noticeable as the loud beats of cardio or the powerful notes of strength training, they're still just as crucial for a well-rounded fitness routine.

Practices like yoga, Pilates, or simple stretching exercises can improve your flexibility, promote better balance, and reduce the risk of falls. It's like maintaining the strings of a guitar, making sure they're neither too tight nor too loose for the perfect melody.

Restorative Yoga

Finally, let's not forget the soothing strains of restorative yoga. This practice, which involves holding poses for extended periods using props like bolsters and blankets, is like a lullaby, calming your body and mind.

Restorative yoga aids in reducing stress, improving sleep, and promoting a sense of well-being. It's like a calming boat ride on a serene lake, allowing you to relax, reflect, and reconnect with yourself.

Remember, the best exercise during menopause is the one you enjoy and can stick with. Whether walking in your neighborhood, lifting weights at the gym, stretching in a yoga class, or cycling in the park, the key is to stay active and listen to your body. With every step, lift, or stretch, you're supporting your body, balancing your hormones, and enhancing your overall well-being. So, lace up your shoes, turn up the music, and let's get moving!

ENERGY BOOSTERS: BEATING FATIGUE WITH FITNESS

Regular Walking

Envision a tranquil path in your favorite park. Birds are chirping, the sun is shining, and there's a gentle rustle of leaves overhead. This peaceful setting perfectly sets the stage for your daily exercise: regular walking. It's as straightforward as it sounds, but the benefits are far from ordinary.

Walking is one of the easiest ways to keep your body active and energized during menopause. Think of it like turning the pages of your favorite book—a simple action, yet each page brings new insights and new experiences. Similarly, every step you take boosts your circulation, strengthens your muscles, and refreshes your mind.

Walking also offers the perfect opportunity to connect with nature, soak up some sunshine, and get your daily dose of

Vitamin D. So, put on a pair of comfortable shoes, invite a friend or grab your headphones and favorite podcast, and head out for a walk. With every step, you're not just moving forward but also boosting your energy, one stride at a time.

Swimming

Picture yourself gliding through the cool, clear water of a swimming pool. It's refreshing, invigorating, and incredibly relaxing. Swimming is more than just a leisurely activity; it's an effective full-body workout that can combat fatigue during menopause.

Every stroke you take in the water engages your muscles, boosts your heart rate, and challenges your stamina. It's like a gentle dance, where the water sets the rhythm, and your body follows the flow.

Swimming also has a calming effect on the mind, helping to reduce stress and promoting a sense of well-being. So, dive in! Let the water lift your spirits, energize your body, and wash away your fatigue.

Tai Chi

Imagine standing in a serene garden, and your body moves smoothly through a sequence of gentle, flowing movements. This is Tai Chi—a form of martial arts that emphasizes slow, controlled movements and deep breathing. It's an exercise form that aligns your body, mind, and spirit, creating a harmonious rhythm that can help fight against menopausal fatigue.

Practicing Tai Chi engages your muscles, enhances your balance, and calms your mind. The movements are like a poem, each flowing into the next, creating a beautiful, energizing narrative.

As you move through the Tai Chi sequence, focus on your breath. Let it guide your movements, filling you with energy and releasing tension. Whether in a class or your living room, Tai Chi can be a peaceful, energizing addition to your menopause fitness routine.

Cycling

Visualize a winding country road stretching out before you. The wind is in your hair, the sun on your back, and beneath you, there is the steady turn of bicycle wheels. Cycling, whether outdoors or on a stationary bike, is a fantastic way to boost your energy levels during menopause.

As you pedal, your heart rate increases, your muscles work, and your body creates natural endorphins, also known as the feel-good hormones. It's like singing along to your favorite song—a joyous activity that lifts your spirits and energizes your body.

Cycling can be adapted to your fitness level and be as challenging or leisurely as you like. So, hop on a bike and let the wheels turn your fatigue into energy.

STAYING MOTIVATED: BUILDING AN EXERCISE ROUTINE YOU LOVE

Setting Realistic Goals

Consider the first time you planted a garden. You didn't expect the seeds to sprout overnight, did you? You knew it would take time, patience, and consistent care. The same principle applies to your fitness goals. It's not about instant results; rather, it's about steady progress.

Start the process by defining what you want to achieve. Do you want to increase your energy levels? Improve your strength? Or perhaps manage your weight? Once you have a clear goal, break it down into smaller, achievable targets. If your goal is to cycle for an hour, start with a 15-minute ride and then gradually increase your time.

Keep in mind that your goals should challenge you without becoming overwhelming. Be compassionate with yourself and acknowledge that progress unfolds gradually. Each step you take toward your goal, no matter how small, is a victory deserving of celebration.

Mixing Up Your Routine

Imagine eating the same meal every day—it doesn't matter how much you love it; eventually, monotony sets in. Variety, as the saying goes, is the spice of life, and your workout routine is no exception.

Incorporating different types of exercises into your routine keeps things exciting and ensures you're working different muscle groups and not overworking any one area. Experiment with a mix of cardio, strength training, flexibility exercises, and balance workouts.

Don't hesitate to explore different activities as well. If you usually go for a run, try out a dance class or a yoga session. If you're a fan of the gym, venture into outdoor activities like hiking or swimming. Keep it exciting and fun, and your motivation will naturally follow suit.

Finding a Workout Buddy

Remember when you were a kid, and everything seemed to be more fun when you did it with a friend? The same goes for exercise. Having a workout buddy can make your fitness routine more enjoyable and motivating.

A workout partner can offer encouragement, share challenges, and celebrate victories with you. They can also hold you accountable, ensuring you stick to your routine even when you'd rather stay in bed. Your workout buddy could be a friend, a family member, or a neighbor.

So, invite someone to join you on your fitness journey. It's like going on a road trip with a friend. The destination is important, but the companionship makes the journey even more memorable.

Rewarding Your Progress

Imagine working hard on a project and not receiving any recognition for your efforts. It wouldn't feel great, would it? Recognizing and rewarding your progress is a vital aspect of staying motivated.

The rewards don't have to be extravagant; they should be meaningful to you and reflect the effort you've put in. A reward could be as simple as taking a relaxing bath after a week of consistent workouts, buying a new workout outfit after reaching a fitness milestone, or treating yourself to a massage to celebrate sticking with your routine for a month.

Remember, rewards are not about indulging in unhealthy habits; they are about celebrating your progress and motivating you to keep going. So, don't forget to pat yourself on the back and enjoy the fruits of your hard work.

In the end, during menopause, building an exercise routine you love is about understanding your body, setting achievable goals, and keeping things fun and rewarding. It's about celebrating your body's strength, cherishing its resilience, and nurturing its health and well-being. So, put on your workout gear, tie up those laces, and get moving.

CASE STUDY: REAL WOMEN, REAL RESULTS

At the heart of every story, every transformation, and every victory, there are real people. There are women, just like you, who have faced the challenges of menopause and discovered the power of exercise and proper nutrition. Their stories serve as a beacon of hope—a testament to the resilience and strength within each of us. Let's delve into the lives of Susan, Maria, Lisa, and Emma to understand their unique paths to success.

Susan's Success with Yoga

Susan, a vibrant woman in her early 50s, first stepped onto a yoga mat out of curiosity. Little did she know that this simple act would dramatically change her menopause experience. With a stressful job and a busy family life, she was no stranger to the anxieties and sleepless nights that often accompany menopause.

As soon as she started to practice yoga regularly, she noticed a significant change in her menopausal symptoms. Her hot flashes became less frequent, her mood swings less intense, and her sleep became more restful. With its gentle stretches and meditative breathing, yoga became Susan's sanctuary—a place to relax, rejuvenate, and reconnect with herself. Today, she swears by her yoga routine and encourages other women to explore the transformative power of this ancient practice.

Maria's Transformation with Strength Training

Maria's menopause journey led her to a place she never thought she'd venture to—the weights section of her local gym. At the onset of menopause, Maria noticed her body changing. Despite her active lifestyle and healthy diet, she was gaining weight, especially around her midsection.

Determined to take charge of her body, Maria incorporated strength training into her fitness routine. She started small, with light weights and simple exercises, gradually increasing the intensity as her strength improved. The results were phenomenal. Not only did she lose the stubborn weight around her midsection, but she also noticed an improvement in her bone density, a common concern for menopausal women. Maria's story is a testament to the power of strength training and its potential to transform your body and health during menopause.

Lisa's Energy Boost from Regular Walking

For Lisa, menopause felt like a heavy cloud, draining her energy and leaving her feeling constantly tired. After receiving some advice from a friend, she decided to try regular walking. She started with short, leisurely walks around her neighborhood, gradually increasing the distance and pace.

The effect on her energy levels was almost immediate. The fatigue that once clouded her days started to lift, replaced by a newfound vitality. Walking became more than just an exercise for Lisa; it was her daily dose of energy, a time to clear her mind and invigorate her body. Her story highlights the power of simple, regular movements to boost energy levels and enhance well-being during menopause.

Emma's Weight Loss with Balanced Diet and Exercise

Emma's menopause experience was marked by weight gain, which is a common symptom that many women encounter. Determined not to let menopause take control of her body, she decided to fight back with a balanced diet and regular exercise.

She swapped processed snacks with fresh fruits, replaced sugary drinks with water, and made whole grains a staple in her meals. Along with these dietary changes, she also started to exercise regularly, mixing up her routine with cardio workouts, strength training, and yoga sessions. The result was gradual, but she experienced consistent weight loss—a testament to the power of a balanced diet and regular exercise in managing weight during menopause.

Each woman's journey is a mosaic of challenges, victories, and transformations. As diverse as these stories are, they all share a common thread—the power of exercise and a balanced diet in managing menopause symptoms. Susan found solace in yoga, Maria transformed her body with strength training, Lisa boosted her energy with regular walks, and Emma lost weight with a balanced diet and incorporating a diverse exercise routine.

As you continue to navigate your own menopause journey, remember that you're not alone. Just like Susan, Maria, Lisa, and Emma, you have the strength, the resilience, and the power to take charge of your menopause experience. So, keep moving, keep nourishing your body, and keep writing your own unique story of strength and transformation. Remember, every step you take is a step towards a healthier and happier you.

CHECKLIST: IDEAL WORKOUTS FOR MENOPAUSAL WOMEN

Incorporate these types of exercises into your routine for a balanced approach that takes into account the changes happening in your body during menopause.

Cardiovascular Workouts:

- Walking
- Cycling
- Swimming
- Dancing
- Aerobics

Strength Training:

- Free weights (dumbbells, barbells)
- Resistance bands
- Bodyweight exercises (e.g., push-ups, squats)

Flexibility and Balance:

- Yoga
- Pilates
- Tai Chi

Bone Density Building:

- Jumping exercises (skipping rope, jump squats)
- Weight-bearing exercises (hiking, stair climbing)

Relaxation and Stress-Reduction:

- Deep breathing exercises
- Guided meditation
- Gentle stretching

It's essential to consult with a fitness expert or physical therapist to ensure that exercises are done correctly and safely.

INTERACTIVE ELEMENT: WORKOUT CHALLENGE

Stay motivated and accountable with our 7-day Workout Challenge! Tailored for menopausal women, this challenge aims to introduce different types of exercises that are beneficial during this phase.

7-Day Menopause Fitness Challenge:

Day 1: 30-minute brisk walk + 10 minutes of stretching
Day 2: 20-minute strength training session focusing on major muscle groups
Day 3: 30-minute gentle yoga session emphasizing flexibility and relaxation
Day 4: 25-minute dance cardio (put on your favorite music and dance!)
Day 5: 15-minute resistance band workout + 15 minutes of Pilates for core strength
Day 6: 30-minute cycling (outdoors or stationary) + 10 minutes of deep breathing exercises
Day 7: Combination day! 10 minutes of walking, 10 minutes of strength training, 10 minutes of yoga/stretching

Note: This challenge can be adjusted based on your fitness level. Always consult with a healthcare provider before starting any new exercise regimen.

To-Do: Try One New Menopause-Friendly Exercise this Week

Experimenting with a new form of exercise can be refreshing and might lead you to find a new favorite workout. Here's a step-by-step guide to help you get started:

Research: Pick one exercise from the list above that you haven't tried before. Look up beginner tutorials or classes in your area.

Prepare: Make sure that you have the necessary equipment or attire. For instance, you should acquire a yoga mat if you choose yoga.

Start Slow: For example, begin with lighter weights if you're trying strength training. If you're attempting a dance class, opt for a beginner session.

Listen to Your Body: The goal is to feel energized and refreshed, not overly sore or exhausted. Adjust the intensity as needed.

Reflect: After the session, jot down how you felt during and after the exercise. Did you enjoy it? Would you do it again? What would you change?

By the end of the week, you'll have added a new exercise to your repertoire, broadening your horizons and diversifying your fitness routine.

7

CHARTING THE EMOTIONAL LANDSCAPE: MOOD SWINGS, SELF-CARE, AND MINDFULNESS

Picture a beautiful day at the beach. The sun is shining, the water is calm, and you're basking in the warmth, feeling at peace. Suddenly, a gust of wind disturbs the tranquility, causing ripples on the water's surface and leaving you feeling a bit unsettled. In many ways, this mirrors the experience of mood swings during menopause—unexpected, sudden, and often leaving you bewildered and off-balance.

The good news is that, just as you would reach for a jacket or seek shelter when the winds blow, there are ways to navigate through the gusts of mood swings. Let's delve into these strategies, specifically focusing on recognizing mood fluctuations, employing calming breathing techniques, and incorporating positive affirmations for emotional stability.

THE EMOTIONAL STORM: DEALING WITH MOOD SWINGS

Recognizing Mood Fluctuations

The first step in navigating mood swings is recognizing them, much like noticing the shift in wind direction at the beach. You might experience a range of emotions—happiness, sadness, irritability, or anxiety—all in the span of a few hours or even minutes.

Keeping a mood diary can be a helpful tool to manage mood swings. Note your emotions throughout the day and any triggers that might have caused the mood swings. This is like keeping a weather journal, noting the changes in wind direction, temperature, and cloud formations. Over time, you'll start noticing patterns and triggers, which can help you better manage your mood swings.

Breathing Techniques for Calm

When a mood swing hits, it's like a sudden gust of wind that leaves you feeling off-balance. One way to regain your balance is through deep, controlled breathing. Deep breathing activates your body's relaxation response, helping to reduce stress and promote a sense of calm.

Try this simple technique:

- Sit comfortably, close your eyes, and take a slow, deep breath in through your nose, counting to four.
- Hold your breath for a count of seven, then exhale slowly through your mouth to a count of eight.
- Repeat this cycle four times.

This practice is like finding a sheltered spot on the beach where you're protected from the wind and can regain your equilibrium.

Positive Affirmations for Emotional Stability

Positive affirmations are like the sturdy lighthouse on a beach, standing tall amid the winds, guiding the ships to safety. They are positive statements that can help you challenge and overcome self-doubt and negative thoughts.

When a mood swing hits, repeat a positive affirmation to yourself. It could be something like "I am calm and at peace," "I am in control of my emotions," or "I am navigating through this phase with strength and grace."

Say it out loud, write it down, or meditate on it. This affirmation will serve as a positive reminder that you are more than your current mood and capable of navigating through the emotional storm. Your affirmation is your beacon of light in the emotional storm, guiding you toward emotional stability.

Remember, navigating mood swings during menopause is not about suppressing your emotions but about understanding them, managing them, and maintaining your emotional balance. You can smoothly sail through the emotional storm of mood swings with recognition, calming techniques, and positive affirmations. Like the captain of a ship, you can learn to steer your vessel, adjust your sails, and make your way through the gusts and gales of menopause.

Remember, seeking help is perfectly okay if your mood swings become overwhelming or affect your quality of life. Reach out to a healthcare provider, a trusted friend, or a support group. You're not alone in this, and numerous resources are available to help you navigate these emotional winds. So, take a deep breath, hold on to your positive affirmations, and know you have the strength and the tools to weather this storm.

SELF-CARE STRATEGIES: NOURISHING BODY AND SOUL

Regular Physical Activity

In the dance of life, movement is the rhythm that carries us forward. As we embark on the journey of menopause, regular physical activity becomes an even more critical part of our daily routine. It's the beat that keeps us moving, the tempo that encourages us to stay active, and the melody that inspires us to keep fit.

Whether it's a brisk walk in the morning, a midday yoga session, or a swim in the evening, exercising daily not only helps manage menopausal symptoms like hot flashes and mood swings but also contributes to long-term health benefits, including heart health and bone density. It's the music that keeps us dancing, the rhythm that keeps our bodies in sync. So, let's lace up those shoes, hit the play button on our favorite tunes, and let the rhythm of regular physical activity guide us through the dance of menopause.

Healthy Eating Habits

In the grand meal of life, our diet is the main course—the centerpiece around which all else revolves. During menopause, maintaining healthy eating habits is like following a well-composed recipe: balanced, nutritious, and satisfying.

This involves a diet rich in fruits, vegetables, lean proteins, and whole grains—foods that provide the nutrients our bodies need without the extra calories that can lead to weight gain. It's about savoring the flavors of fresh produce, delighting in the textures of whole grains, and appreciating the nourishment that lean proteins provide. So, let's gather our ingredients, put on our aprons, and whip up meals that nourish our bodies and delight our taste buds.

Adequate Sleep

In the symphony of self-care, sleep is the soothing lullaby that brings the day to a close. Getting adequate sleep during menopause is like wrapping ourselves in a warm, cozy blanket: comforting, restorative, and essential for our overall well-being.

Quality sleep helps our bodies repair and renew themselves, fosters mental well-being, and improves overall quality of life. It's the quiet serenade that lulls us into rest and the gentle rhythm that carries us into dreams. So, let's fluff up those pillows, dim the lights, and embrace the serenity of a good night's rest.

Regular Medical Check-ups

Menopause, like a less traveled path, can sometimes lead us into uncharted territory. Regular medical check-ups serve as our compass during this phase of life, guiding us through the unfamiliar terrain and helping us to stay on track.

Routine screenings, including mammograms, bone density scans, and cholesterol checks, can help detect potential health issues early when they're most treatable. These checks will lead us through the wilderness; they're the landmark that keeps us on course. So, let's schedule those appointments, ask those questions, and take proactive steps toward our health and well-being.

Time for Relaxation and Leisure

In the hustle and bustle of life, taking time for relaxation and leisure is like finding a quiet spot in a bustling city. Whether reading a book, taking a warm bath, or simply sitting quietly in a favorite spot at home, these moments of downtime are essential for our emotional well-being during menopause.

Leisure activities can help reduce stress, boost your mood, and enhance your overall quality of life. It's the tranquil garden in the heart of the city, the peaceful sanctuary where we can rest and recharge. So, let's set aside those to-do lists, silence those notifications, and take some time to relax, unwind, and simply be.

As we navigate the menopausal phase, let's remember to nourish our bodies with regular physical activity, healthy eating, adequate sleep, and regular medical check-ups. Let's also remember to nourish our souls with time for relaxation and leisure.

Nurturing Your Skin: A Guide to Radiance During Menopause

In the tapestry of aging, our skin serves as the canvas that reflects the passage of time. While navigating menopause, conscientious skincare becomes a vital brushstroke in our daily self-care masterpiece. It's the delicate touch that preserves our glow, the gentle caress that maintains our vibrancy, and the mindful attention that ensures we age gracefully.

Envision yourself gracefully aging, still radiant and beautiful. Menopause brings internal and external changes, and these transformations might manifest as dry, slack, and thin skin. Nevertheless, with thoughtful care, we can mitigate these effects. Nurturing our skin is about embracing organic skincare routines that enhance our natural radiance.

Sun Exposure and Age Spots

Prolonged sun exposure can leave lasting impressions on our skin, especially if sunscreen is overlooked. Aging spots and areas of darkened skin may emerge on the face, hands, chest, and neck. Skin cancer and pre-cancerous conditions may also surface. So, what is our palette of solutions?

Applying sunscreen daily is like painting a protective layer on our canvas. Opt for a SPF 30 or higher product covering all exposed areas. This can diminish old spots and prevent new ones. Regular dermatologist appointments for cancer screening can be compared to preventive conservation for our masterpiece. Early detection is vital, and professional advice for age spots is invaluable.

Bruising and Skin Thinning

Menopause can render our canvas more susceptible to bruising due to declining estrogen levels. To address this, sunscreen with SPF 30 or higher acts as a protective varnish. While it may not thicken the skin, it prevents further thinning. A dermatologist consultation can help you understand the perfect restorative treatment.

Dry Skin and Hydration

Dry skin, just like a parched canvas, can be rejuvenated with a gentle cleanser and frequent moisturization. Make sure to opt for products that contain hyaluronic acid or glycerin. If dryness persists, a dermatologist may recommend specialized treatments.

Facial Hair and Hair Loss

Menopause may bring with it facial hair or scalp hair thinning. Seeking a dermatologist's advice allows you access to the right tools, like laser hair removal or minoxidil, which will be employed effectively under professional supervision.

Sagging Skin and Wrinkles

The loss of collagen during menopause is like the gradual fading of a once-vibrant painting. The skin may sag, forming jowls and wrinkles. Protecting your skin from the sun, seeking suitable wrinkle remedies, and using products with retinol or peptides can help to rejuvenate the canvas.

Acne and Sensitive Skin

Hormonal changes may paint unexpected blemishes on our canvas. Gentle, non-drying acne treatments and fragrance-free moisturizers can help. For persistent issues, a dermatologist might recommend hormonal treatments.

Delayed Wound Healing

In the artistry of aging, wounds may take longer to heal. Recognizing this natural progression is valuable, but seeking a dermatologist's advice ensures our masterpiece remains untarnished.

As we journey through menopause, let's cherish our canvas by practicing attentive skincare, sun protection, and regular medical consultations. Let's also remember to indulge in moments of relaxation and leisure. Self-care, in its truest form, beautifies not just the body but also the soul.

Mindfulness and Menopause: The Power of Being Present

Picture a serene lake, its surface smooth and unbroken. Now imagine a falling leaf, which creates ripples that spread across the water. This is comparable to mindfulness, which is the act of being fully present in the moment, aware of where we are and what we're doing, and not overly reactive or overwhelmed by what's happening around us. During the menopausal phase, embracing mindfulness can be like finding a tranquil oasis amid a bustling city. It's like arriving at a place of calm and clarity where we can tune into our bodies, emotions, and experiences.

Mindful Breathing

Think of your breath like the soft strumming of a guitar— a constant and reliable rhythm always with you. Mindful breathing is about tuning into this rhythm, focusing your attention on the sensation of the breath as it moves in and out of your body. It's the first step towards cultivating mindfulness, the foundation for the practice.

To start, find a quiet place where you won't be disturbed. Sit comfortably, close your eyes, and take a few moments to settle in. Then, turn your attention to your breath. Notice the sensation of the breath as it enters your nostrils, fills your lungs, and then leaves your body. If your mind starts to wander, gently bring it back to your breath. Even a few minutes of mindful breathing can help significantly reduce stress, improve focus, and promote a sense of calm and well-being.

Body Scan Meditation

Imagine you're an artist and about to start a new sketch. Before you make the first stroke, you observe your subject closely, noticing the details, the lines, the shadows, and the form. Body scan meditation is similar. It's about observing your body with curiosity and without judgment, tuning into any sensations, discomfort, or tension.

Start at one end of your body, either your toes or your head, and slowly work your way through each part. As you focus on each area, notice any sensations you feel. Perhaps it's tension in your shoulders, a feeling of relaxation in your hands, or the sensation of your feet touching the floor. The goal is not to change or fix anything but to simply observe.

Mindful Walking

Imagine exploring a new city. With each step, you take in the sights, the sounds, and the smells. You're fully present, soaking in the experience. This is very similar to mindful walking, which is about being fully present in the moment, aware of each step, each breath, and each beat of your heart.

Find a place where you can walk comfortably, free of distractions. As you walk, focus on the sensation of your feet touching the ground, the rhythm of your steps, and the feeling of the air against your skin. Take in the sights, sounds, and smells surrounding you. With each step, you're grounding yourself in the present, fostering a sense of peace and tranquility within you.

Observing Thoughts without Judgment

Much like clouds in the sky, our thoughts come and go. Some linger, some drift away quickly, some are light and fluffy, while others are dark and heavy. Mindfulness involves observing these thoughts without judgment or getting caught up in them.

Imagine sitting by a river, watching leaves float by. Each leaf represents a thought. Some leaves move quickly, and others move slowly. Some get caught in a whirlpool, and others drift by smoothly. Your job is not to chase after the leaves or to stop them from flowing but to simply watch them pass.

Observing your thoughts, like watching the leaves pass, can promote mental clarity, reduce stress, and help you manage the emotional ups and downs of menopause. This practice is like finding a quiet spot in the heart of the city —a place of calm amid the hustle and bustle.

During the period of menopause, embracing mindfulness can be a powerful tool to navigate through the stormy seas. It's about tuning into your breath, scanning your body, walking with awareness, and observing your thoughts without judgment. With each mindful breath and each mindful step, you're cultivating a sense of peace, clarity, and well-being, empowering yourself to navigate the menopausal phase with grace and resilience.

Seeking Support: When to Reach Out for Help

Picture traversing a dense forest. As the undergrowth thickens and the path narrows, the journey becomes increasingly challenging. You realize you need a guide, someone familiar with the terrain who can help you navigate the dense foliage. The menopausal phase can sometimes feel similar to this dense forest. And, just like in the forest, seeking help and support can make the journey through menopause smoother and more manageable. Let's delve into when to reach out for help, how to find a supportive therapist, the benefits of joining a menopause support group, and communicating your needs to your loved ones.

Identifying Signs of Distress

During menopause, staying attuned to your emotional well-being is very important. Sometimes, the emotional changes can grow intense, much like a sudden thunderstorm in the forest. This is when you need to pause and assess the situation. Are you feeling persistently sad or anxious? Have you lost interest or pleasure in activities you once enjoyed? Are you having trouble focusing or making decisions? These could be signs of distress, and you'll want to listen to them. These feelings might be signals that you could benefit from seeking professional help. It's like realizing that the forest has grown too dense for you to navigate alone, and it's time to call in a guide.

Finding a Supportive Therapist

Once you've identified the signs of distress, the next step is to find a supportive therapist. This is much like searching for a guide who knows the forest terrain well and can help you navigate it safely. But how do you find the right therapist? Look for someone experienced in dealing with menopause and its emotional impacts. Check their credentials, ask about their approach to therapy, and, most importantly, make sure you feel comfortable and understood. Finding a therapist is similar to finding a guide who knows the forest inside out and understands your unique needs and concerns.

Joining a Menopause Support Group

Another invaluable source of support during menopause is a support group. This is like finding a group of fellow travelers, each navigating their own path through the forest yet all moving in the same direction. A menopause support group can provide a safe space to share experiences, exchange advice, and find comfort in knowing you're not alone. Whether it's an online forum, a local community group, or a virtual meetup, joining a menopause support group can be a source of strength, inspiration, and camaraderie during this life phase.

Communicating Needs to Loved Ones

Finally, don't forget to communicate your needs to your loved ones. They are your cheerleaders, your companions, and they're always ready to lend a hand or offer a word of encouragement. Open up to them about your experiences, struggles, and victories. Ask for their support, understanding, and patience. Remember, you're not alone in this journey. Your loved ones are there with you, ready to support you every step of the way.

As you continue to navigate the menopausal phase, remember that it's okay to seek help, lean on others, and share your experiences. You don't have to traverse the forest alone. With supportive therapists, menopause support groups, and loved ones by your side, you can navigate the dense undergrowth, find your path, and emerge on the other side stronger and more resilient. So, reach out, seek support, and remember that every step you take is a step toward understanding, acceptance, and empowerment.

Workplace Wellness: Self-Care Action Plan

During your menopausal journey, the workplace can often feel like a battleground where your emotional landscape is tested to its limits. Unfortunately, fluctuating hormones during menopause don't clock out when you start your workday. Hot flashes don't respect deadlines, and mood swings don't align with meeting schedules. Recognizing this, embracing self-care, and practicing mindfulness become necessary strategies for maintaining professionalism and well-being at work.

Acknowledge the Transition

Firstly, acknowledging the transition you're going through is critical. Menopause is a natural phase, not a deficiency or an illness. By accepting this fact, you're empowering yourself to address it without shame or embarrassment. Understand that while your experience is deeply personal, it is also universal—millions of women around the globe are sharing this journey with you.

Create a Comfortable Environment

Creating a comfortable physical environment is a simple yet effective starting point. Dress in layers to manage hot flashes, or keep a personal fan at your desk. If possible, adjust the temperature in your workspace or invest in a cooling gel pillow for your chair. Having cold water on hand can also offer quick relief during a hot flash.

Manage Stress

Stress can exacerbate menopausal symptoms, so managing your workload is essential. Prioritize your tasks, delegate when possible, and do not hesitate to communicate with your supervisor if you need to adjust deadlines or expectations in light of your situation. It's not about reducing your effectiveness but maximizing your potential through strategic planning and self-awareness.

Foster Open Communication

If you feel comfortable, speak to your HR department or supervisor about what you're going through. Menopause is becoming less of a taboo topic, and discussing it can not only educate your colleagues but also foster a more supportive environment. Many organizations now have policies in place to support women going through menopause.

Take Breaks

Regular breaks throughout the day can mitigate fatigue and brain fog. Use this time to step away from your desk, practice deep breathing exercises, or engage in brief meditative practices. These moments of respite allow you to center yourself and can improve cognitive function and emotional regulation.

Seek Support

Building a support network within the workplace can provide a shared understanding and offer an outlet for discussing feelings and experiences. Find a colleague who can be your confidant or initiate a support group for women at different stages of menopause. There's strength in numbers, and collective wisdom can be incredibly reassuring.

Embrace Flexibility

If your job allows, explore flexible working arrangements. Starting later in the day might help if you're experiencing insomnia, or working from home might alleviate the stress of commuting during a difficult time. Employers increasingly recognize the need for flexibility, especially regarding health and well-being.

Practice Mindfulness

Mindfulness can be a haven in the storm, providing a tool to manage emotional turbulence. You can incorporate simple mindfulness exercises, such as focused breathing or mindful walking, into your workday. These practices help cultivate a sense of calm and can reduce the intensity of mood swings.

Prioritize Self-Care

Lastly, remember to prioritize self-care. Whether it's ensuring you have nutritious meals to combat energy slumps or scheduling regular exercise to boost your mood and manage weight, self-care is a critical component of managing menopause at work. Remember that caring for yourself is not selfish—it's necessary for your overall performance and happiness.

Menopause in the workplace requires a multifaceted approach that includes environmental adjustments, stress management, open communication, and mindfulness. By proactively managing your symptoms and advocating for your needs, you can not only cope with menopause at work but thrive through it.

MENOPAUSE AND MOTHERHOOD: NAVIGATING ALL MILESTONES

The tapestry of womanhood is intricately woven with threads representing various stages, experiences, and roles. For an increasing number of women, the threads of menopause and active motherhood are intertwining as more women find themselves raising children while navigating the challenges of the menopausal transition. This time can be marked by complex emotional landscapes, where the dual demands of motherhood and personal physiological changes require a delicate dance of balance and self-compassion.

Menopause is often characterized by hormonal shifts that can lead to mood swings, hot flashes, and sleep disturbances. When juxtaposed with the daily responsibilities of parenting—which may include toddler tantrums or teenage angst—the challenge can be both physically and emotionally taxing. Patience may wear thin more quickly, and the typically inexhaustible 'mother's energy' may wane, leading to feelings of inadequacy or frustration.

In this nuanced season of life, recognizing the legitimacy of your emotional experiences is paramount to your overall well-being. Mood swings are not a failure of temperament but are often a direct result of hormonal fluctuations that are as real as the demands of mother-hood. It's vital to acknowledge that these reactions are normal, and giving yourself the grace to experience them without self-criticism is essential.

Self-care becomes an indispensable part of navigating this confluence of menopause and motherhood. It's not just about the occasional spa day. It involves integrating daily practices that support both physical and emotional well-being. During menopause, adequate rest, even if it means asking for help with childcare, becomes non-negotiable. Nutritional needs may change, and exercise can help manage both mood swings and the physical symptoms of menopause.

Mindfulness practices can be particularly beneficial during this time. They serve not just as a reprieve from the chaos of parenting but as an essential strategy for maintaining equilibrium. Simple practices such as deep-breathing exercises, mindful walking, or even short medi-tative pauses can help regain a sense of control and pres-ence amid the whirlwind of hormonal changes and parenting demands.

Open and honest communication with your family about what you're going through can lead to support and under-standing. Children, even at a young age, can grasp the concept of mom needing a little extra time for herself, and this can be an opportunity to teach them about empathy and self-care. Engaging older children in household responsibilities not only eases your burden but also helps prepare them for an independent life.

Many women also find solace in building a community with others in the same boat. Support groups, whether in person or online, can provide a space to share experiences and tips and sometimes simply have a listening ear from those who truly understand. Additionally, don't hesitate to contact healthcare providers who can advise on managing symptoms and maintaining health during this transitional period.

As a mother going through menopause, it's crucial to remember that this is a phase of life that doesn't diminish the immense value you bring to your family. It is an opportunity to demonstrate the strength of adaptability and the power of self-care, showing your children that every phase of life, even the challenging ones, can be approached with resilience and grace.

Navigating menopause while parenting is undoubtedly a complex journey, but practicing mindfulness and self-care, and with the support of loved ones, it can also be a time of empowerment and growth. Embracing the challenges and joys of this unique intersection allows you to chart a course for yourself and the family that relies on you for love and guidance.

Checklist: Self-Care Rituals

Integrate these self-care activities into your routine to nourish your emotional well-being during menopause. Check off each activity as you incorporate it.

- Mindful Meditation: Spend 10-15 minutes daily in a quiet space focusing on your breathing.
- Aromatherapy: Use essential oils like lavender or chamomile to soothe your senses.
- Reading: Dedicate at least 30 minutes a week to reading a book that uplifts you.
- Warm Baths: Use Epsom salts or essential oils once a week for a relaxing soak.
- Nature Walks: Spend at least 20 minutes walking in nature, absorbing the tranquility.
- Digital Detox: Designate one day or evening a week without screens.
- Journaling: Write down your thoughts, feelings, or daily highlights for 10 minutes each day.
- Artistic Expression: Engage in drawing, painting, or any craft activity once a week.
- Music: Listen to calming or favorite tunes daily. Sing or dance if you feel like it!
- Gratitude Practice: List three things you're grateful for every morning or evening.

Remember, these are guidelines, and it's essential to find what resonates most with you. Prioritize activities that genuinely bring you joy and relaxation.

Interactive Element: Mood Tracker Journal Prompt

Gaining insight into your emotional patterns can be enlightening. Use the following journal prompt to help track and better understand your mood fluctuations.

- Today's Dominant Mood: (e.g., Happy, Anxious, Sad, Optimistic, Fatigued, etc.)
- Possible Triggers or Events: (What happened today? Were there specific events or triggers that influenced your mood?)
- Physical Symptoms (if any): (Did you experience any physical symptoms like hot flashes, fatigue, etc.? Could they be linked to your mood?)
- Coping Strategies Used Today: (What did you do to manage or uplift your mood? Did it work?)
- Notes for Tomorrow: (Any particular tasks, events, or reminders for the next day that might influence your mood?)

Over time, this journaling exercise can help you recognize patterns, identify triggers, and develop coping strategies tailored to your unique emotional landscape.

To-Do: Schedule a Self-Care Day

Setting aside a day that is dedicated entirely to your well-being can have a rejuvenating effect. Here's a guide to help you plan your self-care day.

- Choose a Date: Pick a day you can keep free from work or other obligations.
- Plan Ahead: Ensure household chores or tasks are completed or delegated to free you from distractions.
- Morning Ritual: Start the day with a gentle stretch or meditation. Enjoy a nutritious breakfast.
- Mid-morning Activity: Engage in a self-care activity from the checklist above. Reading, drawing, or a nature walk are recommended.
- Lunch: Prepare or order your favorite meal. Eat mindfully, enjoying each bite.
- Afternoon Relaxation: Take a warm bath, play some soothing music, or nap.
- Evening Calm: Watch a feel-good movie, write in your journal, or spend time with loved ones.
- Night Ritual: Before sleep, practice gratitude. List three good things from the day and set a positive intention for the next day.

By the end of this self-care day, you should feel replenished and more in tune with your emotional needs.

8

SEXUALITY AND INTIMACY: NAVIGATING THE CHANGING TIDES

P icture yourself standing at the shore, watching the waves gently kiss the sand, only to recede and return. This rhythmic dance of the sea mirrors the ebb and flow of our lives, particularly during the transformative phase of menopause. One area profoundly affected by these shifting tides is our intimate relationships. Hormonal changes, physical symptoms, and emotional upheaval can deeply impact our relationship to sexuality and intimacy. But rather than seeing this period as a receding tide, it can be an opportunity to explore new depths, allowing us to uncover different aspects of our sexuality and intimacy that might have otherwise been left uncharted.

THE MENOPAUSE EFFECT: CHANGES TO SEXUALITY AND INTIMACY

Understanding Hormonal Changes

During menopause, our bodies experience a significant shift in hormonal balance. Estrogen and progesterone levels fluctuate and then decline, much like the setting sun that gradually dips below the horizon. This hormonal shift can affect various aspects of our sexuality. Think of it like adjusting the sails on a boat when the wind changes direction. We might need to navigate differently, but a smooth sail is still achievable.

Estrogen, specifically, plays a vital role in maintaining vaginal health. As estrogen levels drop, the vaginal walls can become thinner, drier, and less elastic—a condition known as vaginal atrophy. It's like a garden receiving less water under a hot sun, causing the soil to dry and the plants to wilt. This change can cause discomfort during sexual intercourse and reduce sexual desire, impacting our intimate relationships.

Impact on Libido

The hormonal changes during menopause can also affect our libido or sexual desire. It's like the quieting of music that was once vibrant and loud. Lower levels of estrogen can lead to a decrease in blood supply to the vagina, which can decrease sexual response and orgasm. It's similar to trying to dance without the rhythm and beat of the music guiding your steps.

However, it's important to remember that libido is influenced not just by physical factors but also by psychological and social factors. Stress, emotional changes, body image, and the quality of our relationships can all have an impact on our sexual desires. These various factors are like the different instruments in an orchestra, each contributing to the overall melody.

Changes in Body Image

We also might grapple with changes in our body image during menopause. Weight gain, changes in skin elasticity, and shifts in body shape can affect how we perceive ourselves. It's like trying on a new outfit and not recognizing your reflection in the mirror.

These changes in body image can impact both our self-esteem and our sexuality. We might feel less attractive or less comfortable in our bodies, which can affect our desire for intimacy. It's like our outfit doesn't feel right on our bodies, causing discomfort and self-consciousness.

Remember, though, that we're more than our physical appearance. Our bodies are incredible vessels that carry us through life, constantly changing, just like the shifting tides. Embracing these changes, rather than resisting them, can help us navigate the changing landscape of our sexuality and intimacy during menopause. This transition is about finding comfort in the new outfit, appreciating its unique style, and wearing it confidently.

As we explore these changes, it's important to remember that menopause does not define our sexuality and intimacy. They are fluid, evolving aspects of our identity that can continue to thrive and deepen during this phase of life. So, let's adjust our sails, embrace the changing tides, and continue to explore the vast ocean of our sexuality and intimacy during menopause. The journey may take a different course, but it remains beautiful, full of potential, and uniquely ours to experience.

REIGNITE THE FIRE: ENHANCING YOUR SEX LIFE DURING MENOPAUSE

Exploring New Forms of Intimacy

As the winds of menopause blow, they may stir up new possibilities in your intimate relationships. It's like discovering a hidden trail in a familiar forest—unexpected yet intriguing. The first step on this trail is exploring new forms of intimacy.

A deeper emotional connection, for instance, can add a new dimension to your relationship. Open conversations, shared experiences, and mutual support are the building blocks of emotional intimacy. It's like finding a quiet clearing in the forest, a peaceful space to connect and grow.

Non-sexual physical touch is another form of intimacy. A comforting hug, a gentle massage, and a tender kiss are actions that speak a language of love and connection that transcends words. It's like the rustling of leaves in the forest, a soft, soothing melody that echoes in the heart.

Experimenting with Different Sexual Positions

The trail of enhanced intimacy also leads to the realm of physical pleasure. Experimenting with different sexual positions can add an element of novelty to your intimate moments. Like finding a new dance step, it adds a twist to the rhythm you are already familiar with.

Different positions can offer different types of stimulation, which can be particularly helpful if vaginal dryness or discomfort is an issue. For instance, positions that allow for shallower penetration or more control over the depth and pace can make intercourse more comfortable and enjoyable. Exploring different positions is like finding a dance step that matches the rhythm and mood of the music, creating a harmonious dance.

Using Lubricants and Moisturizers

As your journey of intimacy deepens, you might find yourself reaching for tools to enhance your experience. Lubricants and moisturizers can be powerful allies in navigating the physical changes of menopause. These tools act as a compass and map, guiding you through unfamiliar terrain.

Water-based or silicone-based lubricants can reduce friction during intercourse, making it more comfortable. Vaginal moisturizers, on the other hand, can help alleviate vaginal dryness and maintain moisture over time, like a watering can, nourishing a garden and helping it flourish.

Considering Sex Toys for Pleasure Enhancement

On the path to enhanced intimacy, you might also encounter the world of sex toys. These tools can add a spark to your intimate moments, providing additional stimulation and pleasure. Adding these tools is similar to finding a swing in the forest, adding a touch of fun and excitement to your exploration.

Vibrators, for instance, can provide targeted stimulation, enhance arousal, and even help with issues like orgasmic dysfunction. Using a vibrator is like finding a hidden waterfall in the forest, creating a source of joy and exhilaration.

As you navigate the changing tides of sexuality and intimacy during menopause, remember that this is your unique path to explore. There's no right or wrong way to traverse it. Whether it's through new forms of intimacy, different sexual positions, lubricants, or sex toys, the choice is yours. Like a hiker in the forest, you can choose your trail, explore at your own pace, and discover the beauty in this phase of life.

So, step forward with confidence, curiosity, and an open heart. The path may be new, and the terrain might be unfamiliar. Still, the possibilities for growth, connection, and pleasure are boundless. This is your journey, your exploration, your dance. So, embrace the rhythm, move to the beat, and let the dance of intimacy unfold in its own unique way.

DEALING WITH DRYNESS: PRACTICAL TIPS AND REMEDIES

Regular Use of Vaginal Moisturizers

The onset of menopause can sometimes feel similar to navigating a desert, especially when it comes to managing vaginal dryness. But fear not! Just as an oasis provides relief in a desert, vaginal moisturizers offer a soothing solution for dryness. These products, which are available over-the-counter in forms such as gels, creams, and suppositories, help to rehydrate the vaginal tissues.

Imagine a thirsty plant receiving a much-needed drink of water. The dry, wilted leaves gradually regain their flexibility and color, transforming into a healthy, vibrant plant once again. Similarly, regular use of vaginal moisturizers can restore moisture, reduce discomfort, and enhance the health of your intimate area

The key to success here is regularity. Unlike lubricants, which are applied just before sexual activity, vaginal moisturizers should be used on a consistent basis, regardless of your sexual activity. It's just like providing the plant with a regular watering schedule, ensuring it receives the hydration it needs to thrive.

Topical Estrogen Therapy

If vaginal dryness continues to be a concern despite using moisturizers, topical estrogen therapy could be an effective option. Think of this like how a more potent fertilizer might be used for a plant that needs extra nourishment. Topical estrogen therapy treatment involves applying estrogen directly to the vaginal area in the form of a cream, tablet, or ring. Topical estrogen therapy works by delivering estrogen to the vaginal tissues, helping to restore thinning and dryness.

It's important to remember that while topical estrogen therapy can be a highly effective solution for vaginal dryness, it's not the first line of defense and should only be considered after consultation with a healthcare provider.

Regular Sexual Activity

Lastly, but by no means least, is the role of regular sexual activity in managing vaginal dryness. This might seem counterintuitive, especially if dryness is causing discomfort during sex; however, sexual activity, whether solo or with a partner, can actually help combat dryness. Sexual activity increases blood flow to your vaginal tissues, which helps to maintain their health and elasticity. It also stimulates natural lubrication, helping to keep dryness at bay.

Remember, the key word here is "comfortable." Any sexual activity should be pleasurable and pain-free. If discomfort occurs, it's important to communicate with your partner and possibly consider additional lubrication or changes in sexual techniques. Adjusting to your comfort is like ensuring the river's flow is smooth, steady, and free of obstructions.

Menopause, with its changing tides, can sometimes feel like a daunting desert. However, with the oasis of vaginal moisturizers, the potent raincloud of topical estrogen therapy, and the flowing river of regular sexual activity, you can navigate through the desert of vaginal dryness. These practical tips and remedies are your compass, your map, and your guide, helping you traverse the landscape of menopause with confidence and ease.

OPEN COMMUNICATION: TALKING TO YOUR PARTNER ABOUT MENOPAUSE

Expressing Your Feelings and Concerns

Imagine sitting around a campfire, sharing stories with your companions, feeling heard and understood. This form of open communication is vital when talking to your partner about menopause. By expressing your feelings and concerns, you invite your partner into your experience, allowing them to gain insight into your world.

Sharing your feelings can be like shedding light on a dense forest, making the path clearer for you and your partner. Discuss the physical changes you're experiencing, the emotional ups and downs, and your hopes and fears. Let them know how menopause is affecting you, both physically and emotionally. This is like sharing your personal road map with your partner, marking out the points of interest, the tricky turns, and the smooth straights.

Discussing Changes in Sexual Desire

In the landscape of menopause, changes in sexual desire can often feel like unexpected detours. By discussing these changes with your partner, you're acknowledging these shifts and finding helpful ways to navigate them together.

Be open about any changes in your sexual desire, whether it's an increase, a decrease, or a change in the kind of intimacy you crave. This openness can help prevent misunderstandings and potential feelings of rejection. This conversation is similar to adjusting your compass according to the shifting winds, ensuring you both stay on the same course.

Exploring Solutions Together

As you navigate the menopausal phase, remember you're not alone. Your partner is on this voyage with you, ready to face the challenges and celebrate the victories.

Exploring solutions together can strengthen your bond and enhance your intimate relationship.

Discuss potential solutions to your issues, be it lifestyle changes, medical interventions, or relationship enhancements. Consider seeking advice from healthcare professionals, reading informative resources, or attending workshops together. Trying new activities, experimenting with different forms of intimacy, or even redefining your idea of sexual satisfaction can all be part of your exploration. Embarking on this journey together is like discovering hidden treasures on a map, adding excitement and novelty to your quest.

Seeking Couples Therapy

Sometimes, the challenges of menopause can feel like a tricky knot, difficult to untangle on your own. In such situations, seeking couples therapy can provide a fresh perspective and professional guidance, helping you untie the knot easily.

A therapist can facilitate open and honest communication, provide strategies for managing changes, and help you strengthen your emotional connection. Going to couples therapy is like having a skilled guide on your voyage who can help you navigate the stormy seas and direct you toward calmer waters.

Engaging in open communication about menopause with your partner is like navigating a river together. You might encounter twists and turns, rapids, and undercurrents. Still, with open dialogue, mutual understanding, and shared exploration, you can navigate these waters with confidence and mutual respect.

It's important to recognize that menopause is a shared voyage rather than a solitary experience. By expressing your feelings, discussing changes in sexual desire, exploring solutions together, and seeking therapy if needed, you can ensure that both you and your partner are rowing in the same direction, supporting each other every step of the way.

As we conclude this chapter, let's remember the power of open communication, the strength of shared exploration, and the potential for growth and connection within every challenge. After all, every river eventually leads to the ocean, and every challenge promises growth and a deeper connection. So, let's keep rowing, communicating, and exploring. The ocean of post-menopausal life is waiting, filled with possibilities for continued growth, connection, and satisfaction.

This brings us to the end of our deep dive into sexuality and intimacy during menopause. In the next chapter, we'll delve into how to build a supportive network during menopause, which is a vital component for navigating this transition with ease and positivity.

SIMPLE MENOPAUSE MANUAL | 155

Checklist: Tips for Reigniting Intimacy

Intimacy during menopause might look and feel different, but with understanding and effort, it can be just as fulfilling. Consider incorporating these tips into your relationship to keep the flame alive.

- Open Dialogue: Discuss your feelings and experiences related to menopause with your partner.
- Educate Together: Read articles or watch documentaries on menopause to gain a mutual understanding of this life phase.
- Prioritize Foreplay: Extended foreplay can help with arousal and intimacy.
- Lubricants: Consider using water-based lubricants to combat dryness.
- Seek Medical Advice: Consult a healthcare provider if intimacy is painful or uncomfortable.
- Re-explore Fantasies: Reconnect with your partner by discussing and exploring mutual fantasies.
- Stay Active: Regular exercise can enhance blood flow and libido.
- Relaxation Techniques: Stress can hinder intimacy; try relaxation methods like meditation or deep breathing exercises.
- Try New Activities Together: Bonding over new experiences can reignite passion.

- Seek Counseling: If intimacy issues persist, consider couples therapy or sex therapy.

Interactive Element: Communication Starters with a Partner

Discussing menopause and its impact on intimacy can be challenging. Use these conversation starters to open up a supportive dialogue with your partner.

- "I've been feeling [specific emotion] lately because of the changes in my body. I'd appreciate it if we could talk about it."
- "I've noticed that our intimacy has been affected by my menopausal symptoms. Let's explore ways to reconnect."
- "There are some things about menopause I'd like you to understand. Can we go over them together?"
- "I value our intimate connection, and I believe we can navigate these changes together. What are your thoughts?"
- "I read about some methods to enhance our intimacy during this phase. Would you be open to trying them?"
- "Sometimes I feel [specific emotion] during intimacy, and it's linked to menopause. I'd like your support in managing this."

- "Attending couples therapy might be beneficial for us. Would you consider it?"
- "I think it might help if we learned more about menopause together. Can we set aside some time for that?"
- "I cherish our bond, and I believe open communication is key during this phase. How do you feel about that?"

To-Do: Plan a Date Night Focused on Connection

Use this guide to plan a date night emphasizing emotional closeness and rekindling the spark.

- Setting: Choose a comfortable, intimate setting— at home, a cozy restaurant, or a quiet spot in nature.
- Disconnect: Make it a rule to avoid phones or other distractions during this time.
- Revisit Memory Lane: Start the evening by reminiscing about your favorite shared memories.
- New Experiences: Try something new together, whether it's a dance class, cooking a new recipe, or attending a workshop.
- Express Appreciation: Take turns expressing what you appreciate about each other, focusing on qualities that have strengthened your bond.
- Discuss Dreams: Share your aspirations and dreams as individuals and as a couple.

- Physical Connection: Hold hands, hug, or dance. These gestures can promote closeness without necessarily leading to sexual intimacy.
- Open Dialogue: Use the conversation starters mentioned above if you feel it's the right time.
- End on a Positive Note: Conclude the date by setting a positive intention or goal for your relationship moving forward.

9

BUILDING YOUR MENOPAUSE TRIBE: THE POWER OF SHARED EXPERIENCES AND MUTUAL SUPPORT

I magine standing in a bustling market square. The air buzzes with conversation, laughter, and the occasional spirited debate. Here, in the heart of the town, people gather to exchange more than just goods. They share stories, offer advice, provide comfort, and foster camaraderie. This sense of community, shared experience, and mutual support is vital during menopause. It is a source of strength, understanding, and empowerment, easing the transition to menopause and enhancing your overall well-being.

WHY COMMUNITY MATTERS: THE BENEFITS OF SHARED EXPERIENCES

Emotional Support

Just as a comforting hug can lift your spirits after a tough day, during menopause, emotional support can be a beacon of light in a stormy sea. You feel understood and validated when you share your experiences, fears, and victories with others going through the same transition. It's like finding a compassionate friend in the buzzing market square who listens to your story, empathizes with your struggles, and celebrates your triumphs.

Exchange of Practical Advice

In the bustling market square of menopause, practical advice is a valuable currency. It's like the ripest fruit at the vendor's stall—a treasure to be savored and shared. Whether it's tips for managing hot flashes, suggestions for sleep-friendly routines, or insights on balancing hormones through diet, exchanging practical advice can provide new strategies, broaden your perspective, and empower you to take control of your menopause experience.

Increased Understanding and Empathy

As you listen to others' stories and share your own, a deeper understanding and empathy blossom. It's as if the market square transforms into a vibrant tapestry, each thread representing a unique menopause experience. This tapestry, rich with diverse experiences, contributes to a sense of understanding and empathy that can dispel feelings of isolation, reduce stigma, and strengthen community bonds.

Motivation and Encouragement

In the lively market square, the energy is infectious. The same holds true in a supportive menopause community. Seeing others navigate the challenges of menopause and emerge stronger can ignite a spark of motivation within you. Words of encouragement from your peers can fan this spark into a flame, inspiring you to persevere, explore new strategies, and embrace the change with a positive mindset.

Sense of Belonging

Being part of a menopause community ultimately cultivates a sense of belonging. It's the feeling of being part of something bigger, of standing shoulder to shoulder with others in the vibrant market square. This sense of belonging can boost your self-esteem, enhance your wellbeing, and provide a safe space to express your feelings, voice your concerns, and celebrate your victories.

In the broader context of menopause, the community can be compared to the bustling market square. It's a place of connection, exchange, and mutual support, where each shared experience, piece of advice, and word of encouragement adds another thread to the beautiful tapestry of collective wisdom. Whether you're just entering the marketplace or have been navigating its busy lanes for a while, remember that your experiences, voice, and journey add value to the community. So, step into the square, share your story, and embrace the power of community in your menopause experience.

FINDING YOUR TRIBE: WHERE TO LOOK FOR SUPPORT

Navigating the menopausal phase can feel a lot like exploring a new city. While the experience can be exciting and empowering, it can also be overwhelming. You might find yourself standing at a crossroads, wondering which direction to take, wishing for a friendly local to guide you. In the realm of menopause, this 'friendly local' comes in the form of a supportive community or tribe. Let's explore some places where you can find this community and the unique benefits each one brings.

Online Forums and Social Media Groups

You don't have to venture far to find a supportive community in the digital age. A supportive community is just a click away. Online forums and social media groups are like bustling virtual cafes filled with lively conversations, shared experiences, and valuable advice. Whether it's a Facebook group, a Reddit thread, or a dedicated menopause forum, the online world provides a platform to connect with others, ask questions, and share your experiences from the comfort of your home. It's like having a 24/7 coffee date with friends who understand and support your menopausal transition.

Local Support Groups

Local support groups can be an excellent option for those who prefer face-to-face interaction. These groups are like neighborhood book clubs, bringing together people with similar experiences to discuss, learn, and support one another. They provide an opportunity to meet new people, hear diverse stories, and establish meaningful connections. These regular meetings can become a highlight in your calendar, a space where you can share your experiences, gain insights, and feel a sense of belonging.

Health and Wellness Events

Health and wellness events, like seminars, workshops, or retreats, can offer an enriching and supportive environment. Consider these events like mini-adventures, opportunities to step out of your daily routine, learn new things, and connect with like-minded individuals. Whether it's a yoga retreat, a wellness workshop, or a health seminar, these events can provide fresh perspectives, practical strategies, and a network of support to navigate the transition into menopause.

Friends and Family

Don't overlook the support that's closest to home. Your friends and family can provide comfort, encouragement, and practical help. Open up to them about your experiences, your concerns, and your victories. You might be surprised by their understanding, empathy, and willingness to support you.

Healthcare Providers

Last but not least, your healthcare provider is an invaluable resource. They're like your personal tour guide, equipped with the knowledge and expertise to help you navigate the menopausal phase. They can provide you with medical advice, suggest treatments, and offer referrals to other resources such as therapists or nutritionists. Remember, your healthcare provider is there to support you, so don't hesitate to reach out to them and ask questions.

As you explore these avenues, remember that every woman's experience with menopause is unique. What works for one person might not work for another. It's about finding your tribe—your supportive community that understands your experiences, validates your feelings, and provides the guidance and encouragement you need. Whether it's an online forum, a local support group, a wellness event, your friends and family, or your healthcare provider, your tribe is out there, ready to welcome you with open arms. So, step out, reach out, and find your community. Because in the city of menopause, you're not an outsider. You're a part of the community, a fellow explorer, and a valued member of the tribe.

SHARING YOUR STORY: EMPOWERING OTHERS (AND YOURSELF)

Overcoming Fear of Judgment

Sharing your menopause experience can be a lot like stepping onto a spotlight-focused stage with the curtain just lifted. It's natural to feel apprehensive, fearing judgment or misunderstanding. But remember, your story is not a performance; instead, it's a candid portrayal of your experiences, triumphs, and challenges. By sharing your story, you're not seeking approval but extending a hand of camaraderie to others navigating the same path. It's about speaking your truth, knowing it holds the power to resonate with, inspire, and comfort others.

Inspiring Others

Your story has power. As you share your experiences, the steps you've taken, and the changes you've embraced, you're sketching a path for others. You inspire them to take charge, seek solutions, and find strength within. Every word you recount paints a stroke on the vast canvas of the collective menopause experience, creating a picture of hope, resilience, and empowerment.

Personal Growth

Sharing your story is not just about reaching out; it's also about looking within. It's a moment of reflection, offering you insights into your growth and transformation. You'll see how far you've come, how much you've learned, and how strong you've become. It's a mirror that reflects your strength, your courage, and your resilience.

Building Connections

By opening up about your experiences, you're building bridges of understanding and empathy. You're connecting with others on a deeper level, nurturing a sense of belonging and community. It's about finding unity in diversity, knowing each story adds a unique thread to the intricate tapestry of shared experiences.

Advocacy and Awareness

When you share your story, you're also raising awareness about menopause—a topic often shrouded in silence and stigma. You're advocating for better understanding, more research, and more support. Open dialogue about this transitional life phase is about amplifying the voice of menopause, ensuring it's heard, understood, and respected.

In sharing your story, remember that it's not just your narrative that matters but the narratives of all those who, inspired by your courage, decide to share theirs. Together, these stories create a chorus that can disrupt stereotypes, shatter stigmas, and redefine the menopause experience. It's not just about sharing a story—it's about sparking a conversation, igniting a movement, and transforming the narrative of menopause. So step onto that stage, seize that spotlight, and share your story because your voice and experience matter, and your story could very well be the beacon that lights up someone else's path.

GLEANING WISDOM FROM REAL-LIFE MENOPAUSE STORIES

Coping Strategies

Picture a garden filled with a variety of plants, each adapting uniquely to cope with the changing seasons, the harsh sun, or the biting frost. Just like these plants, every woman finds her individual coping strategies to navigate through menopause. Take the example of Linda, a vibrant woman in her late 40s. When hot flashes started to disrupt her sleep, she developed a nightly routine to create a cool and calming sleep environment. This involved breathable cotton sheets, keeping a fan on her bedside table, and practicing a relaxing yoga sequence before bed. These small changes helped her to manage her hot flashes and reclaim a peaceful night's sleep.

Lifestyle Changes

Visualize a river altering its course to flow around a mountain. It doesn't stop or give up; it adapts and keeps flowing. Similarly, many women adapt their lifestyles to manage the changes brought on by menopause. Consider Sarah, a busy executive. She noticed her energy levels dipped in the afternoon, affecting her productivity. Instead of relying on caffeine, she started packing a protein-rich lunch and taking short, active breaks throughout the day. This shift not only boosted her energy levels but also helped her to manage her weight.

Personal Triumphs

In the journey of menopause, every woman's story is marked by personal triumphs, like signposts in a forest marking the path to a summit. Let's now meet Rebecca, a mother of two. When she started experiencing mood swings, she decided to take up meditation. At first, it was challenging, but she persisted. Now, she meditates for 15 minutes every day. Not only has her mood improved, but she also feels more calm and focused on a daily basis.

Lessons Learned

In the school of life, menopause is a rich learning experience. For instance, when Emma started her transition into menopause, she was taken aback by the intensity of her symptoms. She tried to push through on her own, but soon, she realized the importance of seeking support. Emma joined a local support group, started therapy, and opened up to her family about her experiences. She learned that reaching out for help is not a sign of weakness; rather, it is a step toward empowerment.

Diverse Experiences

Like no two leaves on a tree are the same, no two menopause experiences are identical. Belinda, a professional dancer, was worried that menopause would affect her career. She experienced mild physical symptoms, but the emotional changes took her by surprise. She found solace in art therapy, channeling her emotions into beautiful paintings. On the other hand, Jennifer, a writer, sailed through menopause with minimal symptoms but was caught off guard by a sudden onset of joint stiffness. Luckily, she found relief in aqua aerobics, which helped reduce her symptoms and improve her overall health.

In the grand narrative of menopause, every story matters. Every strategy, every change, every triumph, every lesson, and every experience adds a thread to the intricate tapestry of shared wisdom. So, let's honor these stories, learn from them, and share our own. Because in the marketplace of menopause, our stories are the most valuable currency.

As we close this chapter of shared experiences and mutual support, remember that our menopause tribe is always there for us, ready to share, listen, and support. So, let's keep sharing, learning, and supporting one another. Because together, we are stronger, wiser, and more resilient.

Checklist: Qualities of Supportive Communities

Finding the right support group or community is essential during menopause. Here are some qualities to look for when seeking your tribe.

- Open-mindedness: Members are non-judgmental and open to diverse experiences and perspectives.
- Active Participation: Regular meet-ups, discussions, or events to engage members.
- Privacy and Confidentiality: Respect for members' personal stories and a guarantee of discretion.
- Educational Resources: Availability of reliable and updated information about menopause.
- Experienced Members: Presence of individuals who have already navigated menopause and can share insights.
- Positive Environment: Emphasis on encouragement, empowerment, and positivity.
- Accessibility: Easy to join and participate, whether online or offline.
- Moderation: Guided discussions or monitored forums to ensure the well-being of all members.
- Feedback Mechanism: Opportunities for members to provide input and feedback about the community.
- Diverse Membership: Inclusion of members from various backgrounds, experiences, and stages of menopause.

Interactive Element: Conversation Starter Cards for Group Discussions

If you're joining or creating a menopause support group, use these conversation starter cards to initiate meaningful discussions and strengthen bonds among members.

- "What was your first sign of menopause, and how did you feel about it?"
- "How has menopause impacted your self-perception or self-esteem?"
- "Are there any unexpected positive experiences you've had because of menopause?"
- "How do you deal with the physical symptoms, and do you have any tips to share?"
- "What resources (books, websites, professionals) have been most helpful for you during this journey?"
- "How has menopause affected your relationships, and how have you navigated those changes?"
- "What self-care practices have been most beneficial for you during this time?"
- "Have you tried any alternative treatments or remedies? What were your experiences?"
- "What's one piece of advice you'd give someone just starting their menopause journey?"
- "Share a success story or a moment of empowerment related to your menopause experience."

To-Do: Share a Personal Menopause Story or Experience with Someone

Sharing your story can be cathartic for you and enlightening for someone else. Here's a guide to help you share meaningfully.

- Choose a Listener: This could be a close friend, family member, therapist, or a group. Ensure you're confiding in someone or a group you trust and feel comfortable with.
- Set the Scene: Find a quiet, comfortable spot to talk, maybe over tea or on a serene walk.
- Start with the Basics: Begin by explaining the technicalities of menopause if the listener isn't familiar with it.
- Dive into Personal Experiences: Share your symptoms, feelings, challenges, and triumphs.
- Talk About Your Coping Mechanisms: Mention resources, habits, or routines that have helped you.
- Encourage Questions: Let the listener ask questions to understand better or share their feelings.
- Share Resources: If you've found books, websites, or communities beneficial, then go ahead and share them.
- End Positively: Conclude with hopeful messages or lessons you've learned along the way.

THE SIMPLE MENOPAUSE MANUAL | 173

- Encourage Reciprocity: If they're comfortable, encourage the listener to share their experiences or feelings.
- Thank Yourself: Recognize the courage it took to share and the impact sharing might have on someone else.

PASS THE TORCH OF WISDOM

Wowza! You've sailed through "The Simple Menopause Manual," and now you're practically a menopause-navigating ninja! With all these cool tricks up your sleeve, you're now ready to face the music and dance through this stage of life with some serious style.

But guess what? There are a whole bunch of super ladies out there who could use a guiding star like you. They're just starting their journey and feeling a tad overwhelmed, kind of like how it feels to start a jigsaw puzzle without the picture on the box.

By sharing your thoughts about this book on Amazon, you're not just dropping a review; you're lighting a beacon of hope. Your words can be the guiding light that leads another wanderer to safe shores.

Here's your moment to sprinkle a little bit of that awesome sauce you've got. Let the world know how "The Simple Menopause Manual" helped you kick menopause's butt, and how it can do the same for them.

Click your heels three times, think of that warm and fuzzy feeling you get from doing good, share your review:

Or you go to the link below to leave your review:
http://tinyurl.com/2p864c2z

Thank you so much for your kindness. The wisdom of menopause doesn't have to be a secret club. By sharing what you know, you're helping keep the flame of knowledge burning bright.

Together, we're not just reading a book; we're creating a sisterhood of savvy, empowered individuals ready to tackle menopause head-on. You're not just a reader, my friend—you're a beacon of enlightenment.

Gratefully yours,

Max Hampton

CONCLUSION

The Road Ahead: Embracing Post-Menopause Life

As you step into the post-menopause phase of your life, remember you are embarking on a journey of growth, self-discovery, and renewed vitality. Think of it like the dawning of a new day, bringing a fresh perspective and myriad possibilities. Each day is a new opportunity to embrace your health, nurture your well-being, and celebrate the beautiful, vibrant woman that you are.

Key Takeaways: Recap of Essential Knowledge

As we close this chapter of our shared exploration, let's revisit the highlights of our journey. We started by mapping the menopause terrain, understanding its stages, and decoding its language. We then navigated the world of hormones, explored the symbiotic relationship between nutrition and menopause, and delved into the transformative power of exercise.

We also explored the emotional landscape of menopause, learned the art of mindfulness, and discovered the power of shared experiences and mutual support. Finally, we discussed the shifts in sexuality and intimacy during menopause, and we explored how to navigate these changes to enhance our relationships and our self-perception.

Next Steps: Implementing Lifestyle Changes

Now that you have this knowledge, it's time to translate it into action. Start by implementing small, sustainable changes in your lifestyle. Maybe it's a short walk in the morning, a mindfulness practice before bedtime, or a nourishing meal plan for the week ahead. Remember, every little step counts, and each change you make is a testament to your commitment to your health and well-being.

A Final Word: Celebrating the Menopause Journey

As we reach the end of this book, I want to celebrate you. Yes, you. You, who have made the conscious choice to understand and navigate this intricate journey of menopause. You, who have embraced the changes, faced the challenges, and emerged stronger. You, who are not just surviving menopause but thriving through it. Remember, menopause is not a phase to endure—it's a phase to embrace. It's a testament to your strength, your resilience, and your unique womanhood. So, let's celebrate this journey, honor our experiences, and look ahead with optimism and joy.

Continuing the Conversation: Staying Engaged with Your Menopause Tribe

As we turn the final page of this book, remember the conversation doesn't end here. Stay connected with your menopause tribe, continue to share your stories, and keep learning from the experiences of others. Your community is your support system, sounding board, and cheering squad, always ready to uplift, inspire, and empower you. So, keep the conversation going, deepen your connections, and remember, you're not alone on this journey. Together, we are stronger, wiser, and more resilient.

In closing, thank you for joining me on this journey. It's been an honor to share this space with you and to explore, learn, and grow together. As you continue your menopause journey, don't forget that you are capable, you are resilient, and you are beautiful. Here's to embracing the road ahead with courage, grace, and a radiant smile.

REFERENCES

Carmody, J., Crawford, S. L., Salmoirago-Blotcher, E., Leung, K., Churchill, L. C., & Olendzki, N. (2011). Mindfulness training for coping with hot flashes. *Menopause, 18*(6), 611–620. https://doi.org/10.1097/gme.0b013e318204a05c

Da Silva, T. R., Oppermann, K., Reis, F. M., & Spritzer, P. M. (2021). Nutrition in Menopausal Women: A Narrative review. *Nutrients, 13*(7), 2149. https://doi.org/10.3390/nu13072149

Dąbrowska-Galas, M., Dąbrowska, J., Ptaszkowski, K., & Plinta, R. (2019). High physical activity level may reduce menopausal symptoms. *Medicina-lithuania, 55*(8), 466. https://doi.org/10.3390/medicina55080466

Davis, J. L. (2008, February 20). *10 questions to ask your doctor about hormone therapy during Menopause.* WebMD. https://www.webmd.com/menopause/10-questions-hormone-therapy-during-menopause

Goldwert, L. (2023, May 22). *How to advocate for a Menopause-Friendly Workplace.* Stripes. https://iamstripes.com/blogs/mental-health/how-to-advocate-for-menopause-friendly-workplace

Groves, M. (2018, November 23). *Menopause Diet: How what you eat affects your symptoms.* Healthline. https://www.healthline.com/nutrition/menopause-diet

Harlan, C. (2016, July 6). 8 women who successfully lost weight after menopause. *Prevention.* https://www.prevention.com/weight-loss/g20434709/success-stories-weight-loss-after-menopause/

Harvard Health. (2020, March 1). *Menopause and mental health.* https://www.health.harvard.edu/womens-health/menopause-and-mental-health

Hormone therapy: Is it right for you? (2022, December 6). Mayo Clinic. https://www.mayoclinic.org/diseases-conditions/menopause/in-depth/hormone-therapy/art-20046372

Hot flashes - Diagnosis & treatment - Mayo Clinic. (2022, May 20). Mayo

Clinic. https://www.mayoclinic.org/diseases-conditions/hot-flashes/diagnosis-treatment/drc-20352795

How to cope with menopause symptoms at work | Prime Health. (n.d.). https://www.prime-health.co.uk/blog/how-to-cope-with-menopause-symptoms-at-work/

Jean Hailes for Women's Health. (2023, August 25). *Navigating menopause together: How partners can help.* Jean Hailes. https://www.jeanhailes.org.au/news/navigating-menopause-together-how-partners-can-help

Jkim. (2021, October 4). *A guide to perimenopause, menopause, and postmenopause - Nursing@Georgetown.* GU-MSN. https://online.nursing.georgetown.edu/blog/a-guide-to-perimenopause-menopause-and-postmenopause/

Many women have cognition issues during menopause. (n.d.). UCLA Health. https://www.uclahealth.org/news/many-women-have-cognition-issues-during-menopause

Menopause - Symptoms and causes - Mayo Clinic. (2023, May 25). Mayo Clinic. https://www.mayoclinic.org/diseases-conditions/menopause/symptoms-causes/syc-20353397

Menopause and your heart. (n.d.). British Heart Foundation. https://www.bhf.org.uk/informationsupport/support/women-with-a-heart-condition/menopause-and-heart-disease

Menopause Support and Resources | Hormone Health Network. (n.d.). https://www.endocrine.org/menopausemap/support-resources/index.html

Mishra, N., Mishra, V. N., & Devanshi. (2011). Exercise beyond menopause: Dos and Don'ts. *Journal of Mid-life Health, 2*(2), 51. https://doi.org/10.4103/0976-7800.92524

Montoya, S. (2023, April 11). *Natural remedies for vaginal atrophy.* https://www.medicalnewstoday.com/articles/315089

New York Times. (2021, November 30). Basic biology of menopause: The hormonal transition & what happens next. *The Economic Times.* https://m.economictimes.com/magazines/panache/basic-biology-of-menopause-the-hormonal-transition-what-happens-next/articleshow/88012484.cms

North American Menopause Society (NAMS) - focused on providing physicians, practitioners & women menopause information, help & treatment insights.

(n.d.). https://www.menopause.org/

Np, K. B. R. (2022, July 7). *Natural remedies for menopause mood swings and hot flashes.* Verywell Health. https://www.verywellhealth.com/natural-remedies-for-menopause-what-really-works-2322657

Pacheco, D., & Pacheco, D. (2022, December 15). *Menopause and sleep.* Sleep Foundation. https://www.sleepfoundation.org/women-sleep/menopause-and-sleep

Professional, C. C. M. (n.d.). *Hormone therapy for menopause symptoms.* Cleveland Clinic. https://my.clevelandclinic.org/health/treatments/15245-hormone-therapy-for-menopause-symptoms

Pycroft, L. (2023, October 2). *Building emotional and sexual intimacy during menopause.* Stella. https://www.onstella.com/the-latest/sex-and-rela tionships/building-a-bridge-to-emotional-and-sexual-intimacy/

Rd, M. J. B. P. (2023, April 21). *11 Natural Remedies for Menopause Relief.* Healthline. https://www.healthline.com/nutrition/11-natural-menopause-tips

Regidor, P. (2014). Progesterone in peri- and Postmenopause: A review. *Geburtshilfe Und Frauenheilkunde, 74*(11), 995–1002. https://doi.org/10.1055/s-0034-1383297

Ritual. (n.d.). *Postmenopausal zest: How to cultivate optimism after age 50.* Ritual. https://ritual.com/articles/1-postmenopausal-zest

Royal Osteoporosis Society | 2021.03.22 - What's the menopause got to do with bone health? (2021, March 22). https://theros.org.uk/blog/2021-03-22-what-s-the-menopause-got-to-do-with-bone-health/

Society, E. (2022, January 24). *Menopause and bone loss.* Endocrine Society. https://www.endocrine.org/patient-engagement/endocrine-library/menopause-and-bone-loss

The Health Benefits of Social Support during the Menopausal Transition. (n.d.). https://www.menopausenaturalsolutions.com/blog/social-support

The reality of menopause weight gain. (2023a, July 8). Mayo Clinic. https://www.mayoclinic.org/healthy-lifestyle/womens-health/in-depth/menopause-weight-gain/art-20046058

The reality of menopause weight gain. (2023b, July 8). Mayo Clinic. https://www.mayoclinic.org/healthy-lifestyle/womens-health/in-depth/menopause-weight-gain/art-20046058

Thornton, K. L., Chervenak, J. L., & Neal-Perry, G. (2015). Menopause and sexuality. *Endocrinology and Metabolism Clinics of North America*, *44*(3), 649–661. https://doi.org/10.1016/j.ecl.2015.05.009

Tiffany Athey, MSN, WHCNP-BC. (n.d.). *Take these steps to thrive during menopause: The Association for Women's Health Care: OB/GYNs*. https://www.chicagoobgyn.com/blog/take-these-steps-to-thrive-during-menopause

Upham, B. (2023, October 19). *How to care for your skin around Menopause*. EverydayHealth.com. https://www.everydayhealth.com/smart-skin/tips-for-caring-for-your-skin-as-you-approach-menopause/

Website, N. (2023, July 21). *Alternatives to hormone replacement therapy (HRT)*. nhs.uk. https://www.nhs.uk/medicines/hormone-replacement-therapy-hrt/alternatives-to-hormone-replacement-therapy-hrt/

What causes mood swings during menopause? (2023, February 16). https://www.medicalnewstoday.com/articles/317566

Your menopause stories. (2021, December 23). My Menopause Centre. https://www.mymenopausecentre.com/menopause-stories/

Printed in Great Britain
by Amazon

38005094R00106